WeightWatchers.
She Loses, He Loses

WeightWatchers®

She Loses, He Loses

The Truth about Men, Women, and Weight Loss

KAREN MILLER-KOVACH, MS, RD

BICENTENNIAL
1807
WILEY
2007
BICENTENNIAL

John Wiley & Sons, Inc.

Published by John Wiley & Sons, Inc., Hoboken, New Jersey
Published simultaneously in Canada

Wiley Bicentennial Logo: Richard J. Pacifico

Design and composition by Navta Associates, Inc.

The information contained in this book is not intended to serve as a replacement for professional medical advice. Any use of the information in this book is at the reader's discretion. The author and the publisher specifically disclaim any and all liability arising directly or indirectly from the use or application of any information contained in this book. A health care professional should be consulted regarding your specific situation.

For general information about our other products and services, please contact our Customer Care Department within the United States at (800) 762-2974, outside the United States at (317) 572-3993 or fax (317) 572-4002.

Wiley also publishes its books in a variety of electronic formats. Some content that appears in print may not be available in electronic books. For more information about Wiley products, visit our web site at www.wiley.com.

Library of Congress Cataloging-in-Publication Data:

Weight watchers she loses, he loses : the truth about men, women, and weight loss / Weight Watchers.
    p. cm.
  Includes bibliographical references and index.
  ISBN 978-0-470-10046-2 (cloth)
 1. Weight loss—Sex differences.   I. Weight Watchers International.
  RM222.2.W3252 2007
  613.2'5—dc22   2006036225

Printed in the United States of America

10 9 8 7 6 5 4 3 2 1

Contents

Acknowledgments

Any book coming from Weight Watchers is a team effort, and *She Loses, He Loses: The Truth about Men, Women, and Weight Loss* is no exception. This book compiles the insights, feedback, experiences, and science from dozens of sources, including a number of Weight Watchers leaders and Weight Watchers CEO Linda Huett. The credit for putting it all together in such a masterful and creative way goes to Jodie Shield, who is an MED, RD, and writer extraordinaire.

A special note of appreciation to the couples who generously provided their stories for the "Couples Close Up" profiles. As you can tell from their pictures, these are real people. Unlike the people described in the introductory stories used to open the chapters and the Real-Life Lessons (which I've answered based on an amalgamation of anecdotes and questions from a variety of sources), these men and women gave us both information and inspiration, making the contents of the book come alive. Thank you.

Thanks, too, to the Weight Watchers Global Development Team, including Ute Gerwig, Norma Larkin, Sabrina LeBlanc, Palma Posillico,

Jane Waterhouse, and Sarah Watson, for their insights and contributions as we delved into the Weight Watchers vault of consumer research.

Finally, a note of appreciation to Nancy Gagliardi from the Weight Watchers Publishing Group and Tom Miller from John Wiley & Sons. Thanks for doing all that it takes to turn a concept into a manuscript and finally into a book.

CHAPTER 1

Weight Is Not Just a Female Issue

The statistics couldn't be clearer: the world is getting fatter. Two-thirds of American adults are now overweight or obese. Men and women, empty nesters, and the newly married—the issue of excess weight touches the majority of households in some way. Clearly, achieving and maintaining a healthy weight are a desire and a need for millions of people.

As the world's leading provider of weight-loss services, Weight Watchers has over 40 years of experience helping both women and men lose weight with its comprehensive, proven program that focuses on lifestyle modification. In other words, by following a scientifically effective method that teaches people how to lead healthier lives in a realistic way, Weight Watchers members around the world are achieving lasting weight loss.

Over the years, Weight Watchers has learned a few things about what makes people tick when it comes to weight issues. One of the lessons that has been most illuminating is the gaps between the sexes. The gender gap on the topic of weight is broader and deeper than that on just about any other health-related issue. Despite the huge negative impact that excess weight has on men and women alike, there has not been much medical or clinical research that has tried to understand the differences in how men and women think about weight, talk about their weight-related concerns, or approach weight loss. This book examines what is known about women, men, and weight loss. By exploring the differences, it seeks to provide an understanding of how the genders can join forces to lose weight successfully.

Weight-Loss Research Favors Women

In the world of medical research, men have traditionally been the guinea pigs. Until the past few decades, almost all research on major illnesses has focused on men. In fact, the male-favored gender gap has been criticized as discriminatory, and critics have suggested that it results in better medical care for men than for women. Why have scientists tended to focus their research on men? A key reason is that men are simpler to study from a biological perspective. They do not have the monthly and lifelong hormonal fluctuations that women have; researchers need to control for women's hormonal fluctuations when conducting medical research on them.

There is, however, one area in scientific research in which the vast majority of studies and study volunteers have been women: weight loss. Why? When researchers are recruiting participants for a weight-loss study, the majority of the volunteers are women. In general, weight-loss trials that are designed to include both men and women include 80 to 90 percent women and only 10 to 20 percent men. As you'll learn from this book, this is due to the fact that men tend to be less aware of their need to lose weight, and less focused on weight loss, than women.

The reality is that there are very few studies of weight-loss treatment involving men only in the published medical literature. In doing the research for this book, only three randomized clinical trials (the gold standard in research) done exclusively on men were found. And in the spirit of full disclosure, the condition being treated with weight loss in one of the studies wasn't even obesity—it was erectile dysfunction. The total number of men in the three studies combined was less than 300! That's not even a drop in the bucket compared with the thousands (if not millions) of women who have participated in women-only weight-loss studies.

The lack of male-oriented obesity research is unfortunate because it limits the available pool of knowledge on how best to help men lose weight. Just as women used to be treated for heart disease based on treatments that had been proved effective in men, weight-loss treatment strategies have largely come from studies done on women. Assuming that a man is just like a woman in dealing with weight-related issues is a mistake. Fortunately, Weight Watchers has a great deal of experience in helping men lose weight, and that expertise is shared throughout this book.

Different Sexes, Different Bodies

While the fundamental principles of weight loss are the same for both genders—expending more calories than are taken in—the elements that lead to the creation of the caloric deficit that invokes weight loss are not. Indeed, men and women are different; they are biologically different and emotionally different. Because both biology and psychology are integral to successful weight loss, these differences are extremely important.

The physical variations between the genders require little explanation. The body composition—that is, the proportions of muscle, bone, and fat that make up the male and female bodies—of men and women are quite different. A typical man who weighs 154 pounds has 69 pounds of muscle, 23 pounds of bone, and 23 pounds of fat (the rest is organs, body fluids, and the like). A typical woman who weighs 125 pounds has 45 pounds of muscle, 15 pounds of bone, and 34 pounds of fat. In summary, men are genetically programmed to have more lean muscle mass and heavier bones than women. Conversely, women's bodies are designed to have a higher fat content.

Technically, the definitions of *overweight* and *obesity* are based on the presence of excess body fat (though Body Mass Index or BMI is used to categorize people's weight status—more on this in the next chapter). Here, too, the genders differ. Overweight in men is defined as between 21 and 25 percent body fat and obesity is defined as greater than 25 percent. Overweight in women is defined as between 31 and 33 percent body fat and obesity is defined as greater than 33 percent. Because biologically men are supposed to have less fat and women more fat, even men and women of the same height and weight should have very different body compositions.

Given the physical differences between the genders when it comes to body composition, it's not surprising that body fat recommendations for men and women are different as well. The recommendation for men ranges from 12 to 20 percent and that for women ranges from 20 to 30 percent.

Given their different body compositions, men have a biological advantage over women when it comes to losing weight. That advantage is explored in chapter 5.

Different Minds

Men and women are not only different physically; their psychological makeup is distinct as well. The emotional differences between men and women are an area of great interest. John Gray's 1992 book *Men Are from Mars, Women Are from Venus* caught the attention of the public, sparking discussions of the inherent differences between the genders when it comes to communication, reactions to problems, and sources of conflict.

Psychologists are not the only ones interested in how the mental processes of women and men differ; a great deal of work is going on in the world of basic science as well. Each year, more and more is being learned about the links between mental processes and physical functions, especially as they relate to neurotransmitters. A paper published in 2006 even theorized that the reason men smile less often than women can be accounted for by the way their respective brains are wired. It is well established that our behaviors in the realms of eating and physical activity are influenced by chemical signals in the brain. And while not much is known about those signals at this point, it is likely that there are gender differences there as well. As more is learned about how the brain affects mental well-being as it relates to excess weight as well as the likely impact of gender differences, relevant treatment options are sure to evolve.

The mental aspects of weight and weight loss cannot be overemphasized. The basic physiology of weight loss is relatively simple—in order to lose weight, fewer calories must be taken in than expended. But it is the behaviors—eating, exercise, and thinking—that are at the heart of achieving lasting weight loss. There are clear differences between men and women when it comes to weight-loss behaviors, and this book touches on all of them. Of particular interest are the differences as weight loss relates to how men and women use language, a topic explored in chapter 4.

A Word of Caution

This book draws on a variety of sources to sort out the gender differences and to provide practical insights and solutions so that both men and women can achieve lasting weight loss. Whenever possible, clinical studies from the scientific literature are included at the back of this book. Because, as noted above, there have not been a lot of scientific trials done on this topic, we used additional sources of information as well.

Weight Watchers does a great deal of market research. From focus groups to segmentation studies and consumer surveys, Weight Watchers spends considerable time and money keeping a finger on the pulse of people who want and need to lose weight. Generally, companies doing such research keep close tabs on the results in order to maintain a competitive advantage in the marketplace.

Over the past ten to twelve years, Weight Watchers has amassed a lot of market research that has looked specifically at how the genders differ in the way they think about, talk about, and approach weight loss. In fact, Weight Watchers probably has more information on this topic than any other organization in the world. For the first time, the company has opened its vault of unpublished proprietary information and is including it in this book. As a result, what you'll find is a culmination of clinical and consumer research from which insights and understanding can be gleaned.

It is important to keep in mind, however, that any research—clinical or consumer—summarizes the findings involving a group of people. The reality is that any group of people is made up of individuals who differ. For example, while the research may have found that women are less likely than men to believe that the most effective way to lose weight is to exercise, that doesn't mean that there are not some women who believe this—they're just not as common. Based on this limitation, which is part of any research process, it is easy to develop stereotypes and make generalizations that don't hold true when it comes to individuals. The gender differences explored in this book are based on research findings. Odds are that not all of the findings will apply to any given man or woman.

It is important to use the findings as a starting point for understanding what separates you from a potential weight-loss partner of the opposite sex. With that understanding, you can overcome communication barriers and together, as a couple, find a common ground that will lead to lasting weight loss.

CHAPTER 2

The Weight-Health Connection

How the Genders Differ

The Collins family reunion was right around the corner. Every five years relatives from all over the country—Atlanta, Los Angeles, Boston—congregated in Chicago for a weekend celebration. To kick off the festivities, everybody gets together for a picnic in a park adjacent to a sandy beach right on Lake Michigan. Mike and Ann Collins were making their way to the big event. They had eloped about three years before, so this would be Ann's first time meeting many members of the Collins clan. Ann was extremely nervous about going to the reunion. Even though she had lost some weight, she was still a large woman, and she cringed at the thought of Mike's family seeing her in a bathing suit. She had started losing weight in part because she and Mike were trying to conceive. She knew that obesity was linked with infertility, and after two years of trying, she'd consulted her gynecologist. After several tests, her doctor had concluded that she had polycystic ovary syndrome and recommended that she lose weight to improve her chances of conceiving. Ann had spent a great deal of time finding the right weight-loss program and had developed a keen interest in diet and health.

Mike and Ann arrived at the picnic, and everybody loved Ann. In fact, she felt right at home because from what she could tell, the majority of Mike's family was overweight, too. She spent the entire afternoon getting to know Mike's siblings, cousins, aunts, uncles, and ninety-year-old grandmother. Everyone filled her in on the family history—achievements and physical ailments. She found out that Grandpa John had type 2 diabetes and died from its many complications. In fact, according to Grandma, as far back as she could remember, most of the Collins men have had diabetes. Later that evening, driving back to their hotel, Ann told Mike that they needed to talk.

She said: "Mike, I loved meeting your family, but I'm worried about your health. Your grandmother told me that your dad and your two uncles have type 2 diabetes and your grandfather had it, too; she said that it runs in the family, mostly on the male side. I am concerned because you are built just like those guys—thick around the middle—and I've read that men who carry weight in that area are at a very high risk of developing diabetes."

Mike listened intently to Ann. He thought a few minutes about what she had said. It was true; diabetes did seem to run in his family, particularly in the guys, who were large and had a gut. He said: "Ann, you're right. I really miss my grandfather, and my dad and uncles look so unhealthy. It's time for me to get in shape. I promise you that as soon as we get home, I will call my doctor and schedule a physical."

Weight is an issue for both women and men. At some point everyone with a weight issue must come to terms with the reality of being overweight and how it affects his or her health, physically and mentally. However, excess weight seems to affect women and men differently, as it did Mike and Ann. Like Ann, women often are better informed about how their weight affects their physical health. And carrying extra pounds causes many women to view their body image negatively. That view can affect their emotional health, making them feel down or even depressed. Men, however, tend to be more like Mike. Many guys are unaware of how being overweight can increase their health risk for many preventable diseases such as type 2 diabetes, heart disease, high blood pressure, and possibly infertility. But once men personally experience one of those diseases and someone presents them with accurate information about how weight loss can help, they are usually more than willing to take action to solve their health problem.

This chapter will compare and contrast some of the weight-related medical and psychological issues that women and men face when they weigh more than is healthy. Armed with this weighty knowledge, women and men will have a better understanding of what being at a healthy weight means and how losing weight can have a profoundly positive impact on their lives.

The Difference between Healthy Weight and Attractive Weight

Society seems to have clear definitions about what the ideal woman and man look like, and those definitions translate into a body weight that supports that ideal. The fact, however, is that the ideal weight according to society's definition of what is attractive is not necessarily healthy for most people. And surprisingly, the gap between attractive and healthy is often reversed for men and women.

Today's women often feel that they need to be extraordinarily thin. The icons of beauty that they are exposed

> **Weight Classifications and BMI Ranges**
>
> Underweight: BMI < 18.5
> Healthy: BMI between 18.5 and 24.9
> Overweight: BMI between 25 and 29.9
> Obese: BMI of 30 or higher

to daily, such as top fashion models and Hollywood celebrities, tend to be underweight by medical standards. Conversely, men are likely to see their ideal body as big and broad, like that of a linebacker. The reality is that the body weights that support both the male and the female points of view are not particularly healthy. And that is unfortunate because weight is inextricably linked to health. For health's sake, it's important that both women and men understand that the weight at which health is optimized has little to do with these extreme ideals.

BMI (body mass index) is the globally accepted standard used to classify weight status. Generally, people fall into one of four categories based on their BMI: *underweight*, which is associated with some health risks; *healthy*, the range at which health risks are minimized; *overweight*, which corresponds to an increased risk of several diseases; and *obese*, the point at which health risks sharply rise as weight increases.

You can calculate BMI by plugging your body weight and height into a BMI formula or by looking them up on a chart.

Resources for Finding or Calculating Adult BMI

Weight Watchers: www.weightwatchers.com

National Heart, Lung, and Blood Institute BMI Table:
www.nhlbi.nih.gov/guidelines/obesity/bmi_tbl.htm

National Heart, Lung, and Blood Institute BMI Calculator:
www.nhlbisupport.com/bmi/bmicalc.htm

Centers for Disease Control BMI Calculator:
www.cdc.gov/nccdphp/dnpa/bmi/adult_BMI/english_bmi_
calculator/bmi_calculator.htm

Scientists also use BMI to study the effects of weight and health. When researchers report their findings, they will generally state whether the weight and health connection was found at the overweight

or obese level. For most studies, the risk of a negative health conse-
quence increases as the individuals in the study go from being overweight to being obese.

For most people, the BMI is a good indicator of the amount of body
fat we have, and when it comes to weight and health, excess body fat
is the crux of the problem. One interesting fact is that the same BMI
categories apply to both adult men and adult women. Why? Medical
experts around the world have spent years evaluating the connection
between weight and health. What they have learned is that as BMI
increases above 25, so do health risks for certain diseases, such as cardiovascular disease and type 2 diabetes. And the BMIs at which those
illnesses show up are about the same in men and women. In other
words, despite the fact that men are biologically programmed to have
less body fat than women, research has found that the major weight-
related diseases that affect both men and women occur at about the
same BMI—men get those diseases with a lower body fat content than
women. Take a look at the two following graphs.

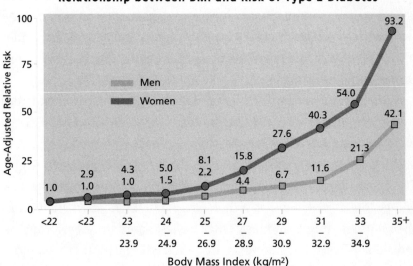

Relationship between BMI and Risk of Type 2 Diabetes

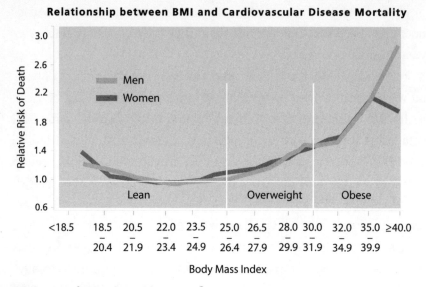

Relationship between BMI and Cardiovascular Disease Mortality

BMI and Waist Circumference: Know Both Numbers

Although BMI is the global standard for evaluating weight status, it does have limitations. While BMI is closely linked to total body fat, it does not provide any information about where the fat is located. And when it comes to weight and health, where fat is carried on the body is extremely important. Studies have found that excess fat stored at the waist or in the abdominal area places people at greater risk for certain health problems, like type 2 diabetes and heart disease, even if their BMI is in the healthy range.

To help compensate for this limitation, experts recommend that waist circumference be included in the assessment of an individual's weight–health risk. For example, there are men with broad shoulders and lean hips who, according to the BMI formula, are overweight. These men have little abdominal fat, however, and their health risk will be low as well. Similarly, there are women who carry their fat in their hips and thighs and have small waists. Same story. Factoring the individual's waist circumference into the BMI equation gives a more accurate picture of health risk than does BMI alone.

How is waist circumference determined? There are a variety of methods out there, but the easiest and most common way involves placing a tape measure around the waist just above the hips while standing. Health risk increases when the waist circumference exceeds 35 inches for women and 40 inches for men.

The bottom line for women and men: know your BMI and waist-circumference numbers. If they are too high, it's time to take action and lose weight.

FROM A WOMAN'S VIEWPOINT
BMI AND WAIST CIRCUMFERENCE: KNOW BOTH NUMBERS

When it comes to gaining weight, most women know exactly where their extra pounds seem to end up—in their rear, hips, and thighs. And several studies have confirmed women's observations. But what many women don't appreciate about their pear-shaped fat distribution is that it puts them at less of a health risk for type 2 diabetes and heart disease compared with guys, who tend to store fat in their middle. However, studies have also found that after menopause, women appear to lose their disease-prevention advantage. That's because hormonal shifts trigger the accumulation of more fat in the tummy area, making women more like men and predisposing them to the same health risks.

FROM A MAN'S VIEWPOINT
BMI AND WAIST CIRCUMFERENCE: KNOW BOTH NUMBERS

While most men are programmed by nature to have less fat than women, they also are programmed to gain weight in the biological danger zone—their gut. Android fat, or apple-shaped fat, is more common in men than in women. Studies have concluded that fat that accumulates in the abdominal area is linked to an increased risk of developing type 2 diabetes and heart disease. But there is good news for guys. Studies have also found that men can significantly reduce their health risk by losing weight.

REAL-LIFE LESSON
Opposite Sex but Same BMI

Situation: My sister and I went in for physicals after our father died from a massive heart attack. The doctor told us that our BMIs were 28, which meant we were overweight. He encouraged us to lose weight because it would help us reduce our risk of heart disease and some other diseases, like diabetes. I am confused about the advice we were given. I weigh 45 pounds more than my sister and look like an average guy. My sister definitely looks overweight. How can the doctor tell us that with respect to our weight, we're the same and both of us need to lose weight?

Strategies: The BMI calculation gets at the volume, or the amount of space a person takes up, and that, in turn, is linked to how much of that space is fat. The calculation uses both height and weight. So while you are taller and heavier than your sister, your BMIs can be the same. Because men typically weigh more than women and have less body fat, it seems intuitive that the BMI cutoffs should be different, and in fact most people would say that a woman with a BMI of 25 would look better if she lost a few pounds, while a man with a BMI of 25 looks thin. The cutoffs used to link BMI and health risk do not take appearance into account, however. When scientists have looked at BMI and health risk in men and then at BMI and health risk in women, the similarities are striking. So from a health perspective, it doesn't make sense to have different cutoffs. Your doctor is right. Your weight is putting you (and your sister) at an increased risk for heart disease. You'd be wise to take his advice and lose some weight. With your shared family history and shared desire to improve your heart health, perhaps you and your sister should work as a team at reaching a healthy body weight.

Excess Weight and Health: Risky Business

It's important for women and men to understand that carrying extra pounds can affect their health. But the reality is that men and women often have very different attitudes about weight and health. While women are usually interested in and concerned about their health and preventing problems, men tend to be less concerned—that is, until they experience a health problem. There's research confirming that men's interest in health appears to lag behind women's. Weight Watchers studies have found that men are less likely than women to take vitamins, scan the media for health-related information, be concerned about their blood cholesterol level, see their doctor for an annual physical checkup, or believe that a positive mental outlook affects their health.

This lack of health awareness is unfortunate for guys, since being overweight puts everyone at increased risk for health problems. That's because certain diseases don't discriminate between the sexes. Four major weight-related problems that affect the health of both men and women are type 2 diabetes, heart disease, hypertension, and infertility. Women can help guys reduce their risk of those problems by sharing information and helping them see the light—the fact that losing weight will lower their health risks. Here's an update on the four conditions, along with the many health benefits that weight loss has to offer women and men.

Type 2 Diabetes

The link between excess weight and type 2 diabetes is indisputable. Even if a person's weight was normal from about age eighteen to twenty-two, adding weight as an adult translates into big risks for developing this life-threatening disease. In a study involving over 37,000 women, researchers found that BMI predicted which women were likely to develop diabetes. Compared with women at a healthy weight, the risk was three times greater for overweight women and nine times greater for obese women. A study that included middle-aged men found that even a minimal weight gain of about 6½ pounds per decade produced more than a sevenfold increase in the risk of developing diabetes.

The take-home message for men and women, though, is positive. Although small weight gains increase the risk for type 2 diabetes, it takes only a small weight loss to reduce the risk. In a study involving about 7,000 British men, a mere 4 percent loss in body weight significantly reduced the risk for developing diabetes. So for a man who weighs 250 pounds, getting down to 240 pounds can result in a substantial health gain. A study involving over 100,00 women between the ages of thirty and fifty-five found that compared with women whose weight remained stable during adulthood, women who gained 11 to 17 pounds after age eighteen had twice the risk of developing diabetes; women who gained 18 to 24 pounds tripled their risk. In contrast, women who lost 11 or more pounds reduced their risk of developing diabetes by at least 50 percent.

Heart Disease

As we saw earlier, since guys are more likely to accumulate extra pounds around the belly, middle-aged men are at a higher risk of developing heart disease than are premenopausal women. But according to the American Heart Association, coronary heart disease (CHD) is the single greatest cause of death for women as well as men. In a study that included almost 90,000 women between the ages of thirty-four and fifty-nine, being overweight or obese was associated with a significantly increased risk of CHD. A gain of even 9 to 22 pounds during adulthood was associated with a 27 percent increased risk of CHD when compared with women whose weight had remained stable.

Once again, studies have found that small weight losses lead to big improvements in cardiovascular risk factors. Researchers estimate that for every kilogram of weight lost—that's 2.2 pounds—total blood cholesterol is lowered by 1 percent, LDL cholesterol (bad cholesterol) is lowered by 0.7 percent, and HDL cholesterol (good cholesterol) is increased by 0.2 percent.

Hypertension

High blood pressure affects millions of men and women in America. Several studies have confirmed that losing a modest amount of weight—5 to 10 percent of one's original weight—can lower blood pressure in both hypertensive and nonhypertensive individuals. For somebody weighing 200 pounds, that means losing between 10 and 20 pounds. In fact, in some cases losing weight normalizes blood pressure among those who have been diagnosed with high blood pressure. And for those taking medications to lower their blood pressure, losing weight often enables them to lower their dosage or go off the pills completely.

Infertility

Although women and men obviously have different reproductive systems, being overweight or obese can affect fertility for both genders. Several studies have found that losing weight can help restore fertility and seems to improve everyone's love life.

For women, being overweight can play havoc with the reproductive hormones. Those imbalances can affect menstrual cycles and may lead to infertility. Obesity has also been connected to women having a poorer response and weaker absorption of fertility drugs. However, weight loss has been shown to improve fertility rates in women, particularly obese women. In one Australian study, researchers put sixty-seven obese infertile women on a lifestyle-based weight-loss program for 6 months. The goal of the study was to determine whether the women could achieve a viable pregnancy, ideally without medication. The results were amazing. Women in the study lost an average of 22 pounds; sixty of the sixty-seven women whose ovaries were not releasing eggs at the start of the study resumed spontaneous ovulation; fifty-two of the women became pregnant (eighteen spontaneously), and forty-five women gave birth. The miscarriage rate was 18 percent, compared with 75 percent for the same women prior to the weight-loss program.

Obesity can affect men's fertility as well. A study of 520 men found that as BMI increased from a healthy level to levels indicating that the men were overweight or obese, the sperm count and semen quality decreased. In addition, several of the lifestyle factors that contribute to heart disease are linked to an increased risk of erectile dysfunction (ED). Smoking, being overweight, and avoiding exercise are all possible causes for ED. Conversely, losing weight seems to help obese men reduce their episodes of ED. One study divided into two groups 110 obese men between the ages of thirty-five and fifty-five who did not have diabetes, hypertension, or high blood fat levels but did have ED. The first group underwent an intensive lifestyle-based weight-loss program, while the control group received general information about diet and exercise. The men in the weight-loss program lost more weight and improved their blood pressure and cholesterol. In addition, about one-third (31 percent) of the men in that group had restored sexual function, compared with only 3 percent in the control group.

Losing weight can definitely help men and women prevent such health problems as type 2 diabetes, heart disease, hypertension, and infertility. The exciting news is that both sexes can reap big health benefits by losing relatively small amounts of weight—sometimes as little as 10 pounds.

FROM A WOMAN'S VIEWPOINT
EXCESS WEIGHT AND HEALTH: RISKY BUSINESS

While women and men share health risks for certain diseases, a few weight-related health problems are unique to women. Losing weight appears to be one of the key ways for women to beat the health-risk odds and overcome those problems. For example, polycystic ovary syndrome (PCOS) is a condition that can interfere with a woman's ability to conceive, and it's been linked to obesity. Since studies have shown that losing weight can improve fertility rates, medical experts recommend weight loss as the first line of treatment for PCOS. In addition, obesity is a risk factor for gestational diabetes. Studies have found that even a modest weight loss of 10 pounds can significantly reduce a women's risk of developing gestational diabetes. Obesity and adult weight gain are also well-established risk factors for post-menopausal breast cancer. In an analysis of a large group of women in Iowa, researchers concluded that preventing weight gain during the childbearing years or, in the case of overweight women, the combination of losing weight and maintaining a healthy body weight during those years, reduces the risk of being diagnosed with breast cancer later in life.

FROM A MAN'S VIEWPOINT
EXCESS WEIGHT AND HEALTH: RISKY BUSINESS

As with women, there are some weight-related health problems that specifically affect men. Losing weight is essential if guys want to reduce their risk. For example, being overweight increases the likelihood that men will develop prostate cancer, and obesity is associated with an increased risk of death from prostate cancer. And the higher a man's BMI, the greater his chances of developing gout. A twelve-year study involving over 47,000 men found that men who gained 30 pounds or more as adults were more likely to suffer from gout. However, those who lost 10 pounds or more since the beginning of the twelve-year study reduced their risk of developing it.

REAL-LIFE LESSON
Yo-yo Dieting

Situation: I'm a forty-six-year-old woman and am about 50 pounds overweight. I know that being obese is not good for my health. I have spent the past fifteen years on and off diets, trying to lose weight. I've lost the 50 pounds at least three times, but I can't do what it takes to keep it off. My husband says that my yo-yo pattern of losing and gaining weight has to be worse for my health than just staying where I am. Is that true?

Strategies: Although a yo-yo pattern of weight loss and regain is not recommended by anyone, it is a myth that it is better to remain overweight than to lose weight and regain it. Why? The health improvements observed with weight loss come quickly; they include lower blood pressure, an improved lipid profile, and an improvement in the way the body handles sugar. As long as you are losing weight and weigh less than you did when you started dieting, those improvements are sustained. No weight loss means no health improvements. That does not mean, however, that the pattern of weight loss and regain is a good thing—especially for your psychological well-being. Rather than working to take off all the excess weight, you might want to try setting your weight-loss goal a little lower. Why not set a goal of losing 25 pounds and choose a weight-loss method with a track record of being sustainable? With that amount of weight loss, you will see health improvements. Then, by focusing on keeping the 25 pounds off for a period of time—6 months is what some experts recommend—you will be in a better position to decide whether you want to stay where you are or lose a bit more.

Lisa and Sam Suarez
TEXAS

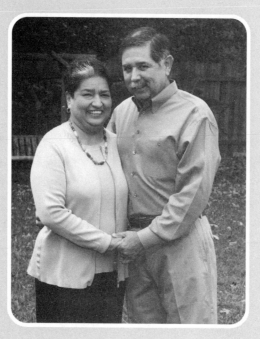

Lisa and Sam have been married for thirty years. They have two sons, Michael, who is twenty-seven years old and lives on his own now, and Sam, who is fourteen years old and lives at home with them. Sam is an IT manager for a federal student loan program.

According to Sam, he's never been especially interested in his health, but his wife, Lisa, has always been health-conscious. "Every year Lisa schedules a physical for everyone," Sam says. Last year at his annual checkup, Sam suddenly became interested in his health. He explains, "My doctor recommended that I lose some weight. My blood pressure was borderline high, I had a fatty liver, and the arthritis in my ankles was unbearable." Another wake-up call for Sam was that both his parents have diabetes. He says, "I've observed what it has done to their lives, and I don't want it to happen to me. I am five feet nine, and at my physical my weight was two hundred twenty-six pounds. Most of my weight is in my stomach, and my doctor told me that that made me a candidate for diabetes, especially if I didn't lose weight."

Sam wasn't sure how he was going to lose weight. Some friends of his at work encouraged him to join Weight Watchers with them. He talked to Lisa, and they agreed it sounded like his best option, so Sam joined Weight Watchers in January 2006. By late February he had already lost 20 pounds and 4 inches from his waist. Sam's blood pressure was within the normal range, his liver tests were normal, and his ankles didn't bother him as much. He says, "I am following the Weight Watchers **POINTS®** Weight-Loss System, and I like how it gives me so many choices. No food is ever off-limits if I plan for it. And I'm walking or riding a stationary bike three to four times a week." Sam says that his energy level and overall endurance have never been better.

Sam attributes a large part of his weight-loss success to Lisa: "She does most of the cooking and shopping. In fact, she bought a handheld **POINTS®** calculator, which she takes to the grocery store." Lisa said that she has had to make some changes in her cooking and menu planning. She says, "We're Hispanic, so a lot of our favorite foods, like enchiladas and tostadas, are usually fried. I've stopped deep-frying and now use a vegetable spray and cook them in a pan. We also eat a lot of salads with lots of fresh vegetables. When we eat out, we look for lighter entrées or we share one large portion."

Sam feels that without Lisa and her constant support, it would have been almost impossible for him to lose weight. Lisa, however, gives the credit to Weight Watchers: "Unlike other weight-loss programs, Weight Watchers teaches you how to eat, and that is something you can live with forever."

Excess Weight: The Psychological Impact

There is no debate; excess weight is bad for your health. But what many women and men don't realize is that it's harmful to your mental health, too. The psychological stress of being extremely large affects both genders in similar ways. For starters, overweight people are often unfairly stereotyped as lazy and undisciplined. There's also evidence that obese women and men may be the victims of discrimination when looking for a job. In addition, studies have found that people who carry extra pounds, regardless of their gender or ethnicity, often have a poor body image and are more dissatisfied with their appearance than people with a healthy weight. As a result of being too heavy, many overweight people often avoid social situations and spend more time alone that do healthy-weight people.

While excess weight negatively affects the psychological well-being of both genders, it seems to take a greater emotional toll on women. Studies have found that women are more likely than men to be dissatisfied with their weight and overall body image. And most women's dissatisfaction with their weight starts early in life and lasts throughout adulthood. Why? The answer lies, at least in part, in our cultural obsession with female thinness. Weight Watchers researchers often hear women say that they feel that others judge them more on their appearance (how thin and attractive they are) than on who they are and what they are capable of doing. Where do women get that belief? The media is a key source. Most of the beautiful women featured in magazines or on the big screen are extraordinarily thin, and for many women, extraordinary thinness becomes their standard of beauty.

This seems to be primarily a woman's issue. In a study in which men and women were asked to evaluate ideal body shapes and assess how they thought their bodies compared with their ideals, men were found to be generally satisfied. In contrast, the women consistently saw themselves as being heavier than their ideal and expressed a desire to be thinner.

Unfortunately, this extremely thin waif figure is unrealistic (and unhealthy!) and cannot be achieved by most women. As a result, many women's self-esteem plummets, and women develop a negative body image—both factors that have been linked to depression.

Although body image is primarily a woman's issue, excess weight affects men's mental well-being, too. Studies have found that the major difference is that men tend to perceive a negative image of their weight at a later age than women do. Research shows that men typically spend their early years satisfied with their weight and body image. It's not until later in adulthood, when they've often gained a substantial amount of weight, that guys' body image takes a nosedive. In a study that evaluated this phenomenon, researchers looked at three generations of family members (undergraduate students, their parents, and their grandparents). They found that the men's satisfaction with their body image decreased with age, while the women's satisfaction remained relatively low throughout the adult years.

Why do men appear to have a delayed negative reaction to their body image compared with women? Some research suggests that men are less likely to see themselves as being judged on appearance and more likely to see themselves as being judged on their personal achievements, such as their career title or their athletic performance. As a result, many guys aren't as bothered by their weight until later in life, when it becomes a health problem.

That said, it does appear that men's perceptions may be changing and the gender gap may be changing when it comes to body image. Over the past few years, guys have been exposed to more advertising campaigns featuring younger male models with sculpted bodies and six-pack abs. Therefore, men's bodies are under greater scrutiny and there seems to be a growing trend for guys to aspire to an unrealistic ideal Adonis standard. Weight Watchers research has also picked up on this trend. After conducting years of weight-loss research on both men and women, only now do Weight Watchers surveys find that younger men are saying that their primary reason for losing weight is appearance.

The reality is that carrying extra pounds has negative psychological consequences. Being overweight often makes both women and men feel bad about how they look and may even lead to depression, especially for women. But there is no need for anyone to despair. The good news is that losing weight can help both women and men look and feel better. There is plenty of research out there to prove it. For starters, losing weight improves perceptions of body image and can alleviate depression. In a randomized clinical trial, researchers found that women assigned to participate in Weight Watchers for twelve weeks lost significantly more weight and experienced improvement in their body satisfaction, mood, self-worth, and other quality-of-life measures when compared with a control group (who were assigned to an exercise group). Another Weight Watchers study found that simply *trying* to lose weight improved mood independently of the amount of weight lost or the length of the program. Why might that be? The researchers concluded that the psychological benefits of weight-management programs that include group support, as Weight Watchers does, extend beyond the number of pounds people lose. Finally, while losing weight can bolster body image, keeping the weight off may offer even greater psychological benefits. In a study of people in the National Weight Control Registry (a database of women and men who have lost at least 30 pounds and kept it off for at least 1 year), more than 85 percent reported that their quality of life, mood, and self-confidence had improved since losing weight. So the take-away message for women and men is that taking weight off and keeping it off are linked to greater feelings of happiness.

FROM A WOMAN'S VIEWPOINT
EXCESS WEIGHT: THE PSYCHOLOGICAL IMPACT

Race seems to play a role in how women view themselves in relation to their weight. According to the most recent national weight statistics, there are more overweight and obese African American women than white or Hispanic women. Yet despite that fact, studies have found that black women often report being more satisfied with their appearance and tend to prefer a larger body size than women in other ethnic groups. Why do African American women seem to have a greater acceptance of a larger body image? Part of the answer may be that African American men are more accepting of them. Studies have found that black men are more likely than white or Hispanic men to accept greater variations in the body size of a woman they consider beautiful.

FROM A MAN'S VIEWPOINT
EXCESS WEIGHT: THE PSYCHOLOGICAL IMPACT

Race also plays a role in how men view themselves, as well as how they view other men. Despite the fact that the most recent national weight statistics indicate that there are more obese African American and Hispanic men than obese white men, studies have found that white men tend to be more dissatisfied with their appearance. Why the disparity? Studies reveal that society tends to view obese black men more positively than it views obese white men. One study found that large black men are often viewed as healthy and athletic while obese white men were more likely to be seen as unhealthy and unfit. The reality is that all men carrying excess weight should take the problem seriously.

REAL-LIFE LESSON
Weight Is Getting a Wife Down

Situation: My wife has put on about 25 pounds over the last few years. I would describe her as pleasingly plump but not obese. Her weight doesn't bother me, but it bothers her a lot. In fact, it has gotten to the point where it is affecting our social life. We rarely go out with friends or to social events anymore. And she's always saying negative things about herself such as, "I'm too fat to go to that party" or "I hate the way I look!" I'm a little overweight, too, but I try not to let it get me down. Is there anything I can do to help my wife?

Strategies: The single greatest gift you can give your wife is a sincere offer to lose weight with her. Clearly she is unhappy with her current weight. Providing encouraging words to help her get started on a weight-loss program will help tremendously, but joining her in the process will have an even bigger impact. Working as a team to make wise food choices, engage in physical activity, learn positive thinking skills, and support each other's challenges and successes can provide your wife with the boost she needs to emerge from the darkness that her current situation has created. And by helping your wife, you'll help yourself, too!

Wrapping Things Up

Excess weight affects the lives of both women and men. Being overweight has health consequences affecting both physical and mental well-being. The first step is to separate the definition of an attractive weight from the definition of a healthy weight. The second step is to see how you and your partner measure up when it comes to being at a healthy weight. Based on that reality check, you can make an informed decision about the need to lose weight. And if losing weight is the reasonable answer, be assured that doing so can provide both men and women with significant health benefits and an improved quality of life.

- A weight that society considers attractive is typically not the same as a weight that scientists consider healthy. Doctors and researchers use a measurement called the body mass index (BMI) to determine weight status. The BMI ranges are the same for women and men. They can easily be calculated using a formula that analyzes height and weight or they can be determined by consulting one of many Web sites. A limitation of the BMI is that it can't determine whether excess body fat is stored in the danger zone—the belly. Adding waist circumference to the BMI provides a better assessment of whether or not weight loss is needed.

- Carrying extra weight predisposes both women and men to health problems such as type 2 diabetes, heart disease, hypertension, and infertility. In addition, each of the sexes has a unique set of weight-related health risks. But the good news is that losing weight—even as little as 10 pounds—can help reduce the risks and/or improve existing health issues.

- Being overweight has a psychological impact on women and men of all ethnic backgrounds. Women tend to adopt a negative body image earlier in life than men do. Women often feel that they are judged more on their appearance than on their talent or achievements. The typical male experience is different. Men generally start out with a positive body image, but as the years go by and the pounds go up, the body image becomes increasingly negative. And because men are more likely than women to feel that they are judged more on performance and less on appearance, they tend to have fewer negative emotions related to their weight.

Let's Talk!

Before deciding that losing weight is the right course of action for you, it's important to assess your risks and realize your weight-loss advantages. To explore this area, spend a few minutes thinking about the following questions:

1. What is your body mass index (BMI)? What is your waist circumference? How do they compare with what the experts say is a healthy weight and waist circumference?

2. Are you experiencing or at high risk for any weight-related health problems?

3. Does your weight affect your mood and how you feel about your body?

CHAPTER 3

When and How
the Mirror Lies

It's Saturday night and Donna and Steve are getting dressed to go to a party. Donna has spent over 45 minutes riffling through her closet for something to wear. She's tried on at least fifteen different outfits, but everything feels too tight. As she's trying to squeeze into a pair of black slacks, she looks desperately into the mirror. She says, "I am so fat! I've got to go on a diet! I need to lose at least twenty pounds!"

Meanwhile, Steve, who has waited until the last minute to get dressed, rummages quickly through his dresser drawer and pulls out an old sweater. He wrestles with it for a few minutes trying to get it over his stomach; it feels rather snug, but it goes on. He takes a quick look at himself in the mirror and says, "Hey, this fits! Guess I'm still in OK shape."

Here's something that you didn't know about Donna and Steve: Steve has a BMI of 32, while Donna's is 26. (See chapter 2 for more on

BMI.) Bottom line: Steve is obese and Donna is just a little overweight. While they are looking at themselves in the same bathroom mirror, they see their bodies very differently. The fact is that they have very different perspectives—and both are a bit off. One thing they do share is that their perceptions of their weight, along with their reactions, mirror how the majority of men and women view themselves. Women tend to look at themselves and come up with a more realistic yet often overly harsh assessment of their weight. It is not uncommon for a woman at a healthy weight to believe that she needs to lose weight. Many men, on the other hand, spend less time looking at and thinking about their bodies, and it is not uncommon for them to assess their weight as healthy when in fact it is not.

Weight awareness is one of the major weight gaps between men and women. This chapter provides insights into how women and men perceive body weight and explore how their different perspectives can affect the decision to lose weight.

Who's More Overweight, Women or Men?

Since weight is often thought of as a woman's issue, most of us would be tempted to answer that question by saying women are. But there are actually more overweight men in the US than overweight women. According to the latest national statistics, 71 percent of adult men and 62 percent of adult women are overweight. When it comes to obesity, the news is different—there are more obese women than obese men.

The landscape when it comes to who's more obese seems to be changing, however. The rate among adult women is about 33 percent and has stayed relatively steady for several years. And although there are fewer obese men—the current rate is 31 percent—that number is on the rise. For example, in 1999 only 27.5 percent of men were obese. Men now make up one of the fastest-growing groups of weight gainers in our society (children are another).

Why are men more likely to be overweight than women? While several factors undoubtedly account for the difference, the gender gap when it comes to self-assessment may play an important role. Women are more likely than men to identify themselves as overweight, while men are more likely to remain unaware of the status of their weight.

FROM A WOMAN'S VIEWPOINT
WHO'S MORE OVERWEIGHT, WOMEN OR MEN?

Women are not in wonderland when they're in front of the looking glass. Researchers have confirmed that compared with men, women are more accurate in assessing the status of their weight. They seem to be able to quickly pinpoint when and where they are accumulating body fat and are faster to acknowledge a need to lose weight. And if a woman is actively gaining weight or is already overweight or obese, that finely tuned ability to see body fat is good news. But it can have a dark side, too.

It's no secret that our society values thinness in women. Underweight women routinely grace the covers of popular women's magazines and star in the latest Hollywood films. But the reality is that being underweight also carries health risks. The constant exposure to too-thin women may create an environment in which a woman who is already at a healthy weight may feel the need to lose weight and a woman who is overweight may overestimate the amount of weight she needs to lose. Indeed, in a woman's mind, there tends to be a mix-up between the body weight that is desirable for good health and the one that is deemed desirable for appearance. Surveys have found that this is particularly true for young and middle-aged women, who are often more likely to consider themselves overweight even when their weight is within the recommended range.

FROM A MAN'S VIEWPOINT
WHO'S MORE OVERWEIGHT, WOMEN OR MEN?

Are these shirt collars getting tight or did the dry cleaner shrink them? Studies have found that many men's ability to assess their weight status is less finely tuned than women's. Why might this be? The reason could be in part that compared with women, the majority of men have less practice analyzing their bodies and, in turn, their weight. Other than shaving, brushing their teeth, and buying new clothes, men typically don't spend much time in front of a mirror. Whereas a woman can easily spend 45 to 60 minutes getting ready for her day—in the shower, styling her hair, applying cosmetics, and dressing—men tend to spend a fraction of that time in their daily ritual. Let's be honest— the amount of face time the genders spend in front of a mirror (especially a full-length one) is very different.

Another factor that can skew a guy's self-assessment skills when it comes to his weight is our societal view of what men are supposed to look like. Just as our culture values very thin women, it also values large, strong men. A comment like "He looks like a linebacker" is a compliment for most guys and an aspiration of many young men. So when some guys do take a good look at their bodies they see themselves as big rather than overweight.

There's another irony when it comes to men, women, and their perceptions of weight. Just as women confuse the ideal-for-appearance body with the ideal-for-health body, so do men—but the opposite way.

Fat Detectors

Although women are more likely than men to assess their weight status accurately, gender isn't the only factor that influences how weight is judged. A 2002 study conducted by researchers at the Pennington Biomedical Research Center discovered that race, BMI, education, and income also play a role. Being Caucasian, lean, or well educated or having a higher income is associated with a greater likelihood of correctly assessing one's weight status.

One study of over 29,000 men and women found that a considerable number of overweight men were satisfied with their current weight and so were not making any attempt to reduce it. In other words, men are likely to believe that the weight that is healthy for them is greater than what research has shown it to be. Since men are without an awareness of what a healthy weight is, it's no wonder that the number of overweight and obese men is on the rise.

REAL-LIFE LESSON

Encouraging Husbands to Lose Weight

Situation: My husband knows he is overweight, so why won't he do something about it?

Strategies: Although I don't know your husband, I do know that most men share the trait of being problem-solvers. Because most guys are results-oriented and performance-driven, the key to encouraging your husband to lose weight is to help him discover that he has a problem he can fix. You might want to try helping him identify a weight-related problem that he'd be motivated to do something about, (because the weight itself is probably not a problem worth fixing in his eyes). Examples include getting him to make an appointment for a long-needed visit to the doctor to see if his blood pressure and triglycerides are elevated or if his nagging back pain is the result of carrying too much weight. Or you might suggest that he needs to go shopping for bigger clothes because the ones in his closet don't fit anymore (doing his shopping for him is not fair). Helping your husband realize that he has a real problem is the first step in helping him make the decision to lose weight.

How Couples Think and Feel about Their Weight

A study sponsored by Weight Watchers found that men and women who described themselves as overweight tended to differ in how often they thought about their weight and in their emotional reactions to those thoughts. The women in the study reported thinking about their weight more frequently than the men. When asked what events would trigger thoughts about their weight, the women identified a number of diverse things. For example, women closely linked weight and clothing, saying that getting dressed in the morning, getting undressed at night, and buying clothes made them think about their weight. In addition, the women said that they thought about their weight when they were in the public eye, such as when they attended celebrations of special events. Finally, experiences of physical discomfort (feeling tired or too hot, having feet that hurt or other aches and pains) or emotional distress (a low self-image, a lack of self-confidence, or depression) triggered thoughts about their weight. When asked about their emotional responses to their thoughts about their weight, the women were more likely than the men to say that the thoughts elicited negative emotions like disgust or anxiety.

When asked the same series of questions, men identified fewer trigger times when they thought about weight. They shared with women the association with clothes, describing getting dressed, undressed, and shopping for clothes as times when they thought about their weight. Men also described linking weight to physical health, saying that experiencing physical limitations like being out of breath or feeling fatigued and being told by their doctor that they had a weight-related medical condition made them think about their weight status. Interestingly, men did not link being out in public or times of emotional distress to thoughts about their weight. When asked to describe the emotional response to thoughts about their weight, the men were more likely to speak in terms of being "bothered," whereas the women expressed deeper negative emotions.

This study shows another dimension of the gender weight gap. In addition to the differences in self-assessment regarding weight status, women and men differ in their reactions to the weight once the awareness is there. By thinking about their weight more often and having a stronger negative reaction to it, it follows that women are more likely than men to take action to lose weight. Conversely, the tendency of men to have less frequent thoughts about their weight and to react to those thoughts with milder feelings, such as annoyance or bother, helps us understand why many guys may place a lower priority on weight loss.

FROM A WOMAN'S VIEWPOINT
HOW COUPLES THINK AND FEEL ABOUT THEIR WEIGHT

Not only do women think about their weight, but they also care what others think—sometimes too much. Believing that they are being judged on the basis of their weight is largely a female phenomenon. In a Weight Watchers survey, women talked about their public persona and its contribution to a poor self-image—not looking as good as they would like and not feeling good about themselves. In fact, some of the women admitted that they were depressed by their weight and embarrassed to be seen in a bathing suit, two factors that never came up among the men who took part in the survey.

FROM A MAN'S VIEWPOINT
HOW COUPLES THINK AND FEEL ABOUT THEIR WEIGHT

When it comes to their weight, men spend less time thinking about it—until their health is negatively affected, as with a diagnosis of high blood pressure, elevated cholesterol, or diabetes. Men also appear to have fewer emotional connections with their weight. Why? Weight Watchers research suggests that men are more likely to see their excess weight as a matter of genetics or the way they were fed growing up. In other words, men tend to see their weight as inevitable, not something to be ashamed of.

REAL-LIFE LESSON
Weight-Conscious Wives

Situation: I do not understand why my wife and daughter are so focused on their weight and seem to blame their weight when things don't go right in their lives. For example, my daughter recently did not get a job that she wanted and was convinced that it was because of her weight (she's only slightly overweight). My wife twisted her ankle recently and said that if she weighed what she should, it would never have happened. Even when they are losing weight, they can't seem to get past blaming their weight. What can I say to help them see past the weight and understand that sometimes things just don't go your way?

Strategies: The first thing you need to understand is that many women view the world through a weight lens. That mind-set probably stems from the fact that women tend to think about their weight more often and are usually more emotional about it than men. So it's not uncommon for women—including your wife and your daughter—to blame problems on their weight. I hear it all the time. Tired after being up all night with the baby? Must be the weight. Feeling blue because a deadline at work was missed? Again, it's the weight. Can't find the right outfit for an upcoming event? Bingo! Guys who understand this can help the women in their lives reframe the factual reasons behind the negative feelings. Lack of sleep, unrealistic demands at work, bad luck, and the frustration of shopping for clothes—not one's weight—are more likely to be at the root of such hassles. Helping your girls expand beyond their weight the reasons why everyday obstacles crop up can help them not only focus less on their weight but also deal more effectively with those issues as they occur.

Randy and Regina Jones
ILLINOIS

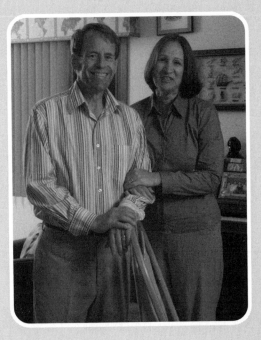

Randy and Regina have been married for 22 years. They have two daughters, twenty-year-old Jessica, who's away at college, and fifteen-year-old Amanda. Randy works as a quality manager for a furniture manufacturer. His job requires him to travel frequently and spend many evenings dining with clients. Regina works full-time as a traffic specialist for a health care manufacturer. Although her job doesn't require her to travel as much as Randy's job, she does work long hours.

Randy feels that all his life he has been on the heavy side, but he never thought of himself as overweight. "In high school I started playing soccer and really slimmed down. During my college years, I was in terrific shape because I went to a U.S. Merchant Marine Academy and we worked out all the time." Randy believes that he started putting on weight and noticing it after getting married and having children. "I was really starting to slow down, and I found myself getting short of breath from simple things like climbing stairs. Being heavy didn't bother me that much, but it really bothered Regina. She started making me go for annual physicals with a doctor." After his first exam, Randy discovered that his weight had skyrocketed to 316 pounds and that his blood pressure and cholesterol were high. His doctor put him on medications and encouraged him to lose weight.

Regina never had a weight problem until after the birth of their second daughter. "I tried several times to lose the extra thirty pounds I had put on from carrying Amanda. Once I came very close to my prepregnancy weight, but I eventually gained back all the weight." Regina said she was always self-conscious about her weight.

In 2003 Randy's doctor gave him some alarming news. "He told me that if I didn't lose weight it was no longer a matter of if but when I would get diabetes." This was the trigger Randy needed to shed his extra pounds. He asked his wife what he should do, and Regina recommended Weight Watchers: Randy joined that week. "My mom had been on Weight Watchers when I was a kid. I was amazed at how much the program had changed. It was way more flexible, and there were more guys in the program." Randy started with the Flex Plan, which focuses on portion control, than decided to switch to the Core Plan, which focuses on foods with a low energy density. His weight seemed to melt off. And he found that Weight Watchers was easy to follow even when he was traveling. "I always make sure that I order a salad and some type of fish— something I love but we rarely eat when I'm at home."

Inspired by Randy's weight loss success, Regina joined Weight Watchers a few months after her husband. "I came to the conclusion that the best way for Randy to continue losing weight was for me to join Weight Watchers so we could then help each other. I never had success keeping weight off on my own, and I didn't want Randy to fail."

Currently Randy and Regina have lost their excess weight and are lifetime Weight Watchers members. Randy explains, "We love the program! Losing weight together has helped us both be healthier and happier. We've made so many new friends from going to Weight Watchers meetings. We couldn't imagine how people lose weight on their own." They both follow the Flex Plan now, and their eating habits have rubbed off on their daughters. Randy said, "It's funny. I was so huge before I lost weight, but I just never realized it. My youngest daughter once told me she is so happy that I lost weight because now she can reach her arms around me and give me a real hug!"

Who's Trying to Lose Weight?

There is no sex discrimination when it comes to being overweight—it is an issue for both women and men. With two-thirds of adults weighing more than they should, the need to take action is enormous. Fortunately, there are signs that the gap between the genders is narrowing when it comes to who is taking up the weight-loss challenge.

The Behavioral Risk Factor Surveillance System (BRFSS) is a survey by the Centers for Disease Control and Prevention that tracks what's happening in the United States on a variety of health-related topics. One of the areas that the survey deals with is weight loss. In 1989, 23 percent of the men and 40 percent of the women reported that they were attempting to lose weight. Those numbers had risen to 29 percent and 44 percent when the question was asked again in 1996. The question was asked most recently in 2000, when 31 percent of the men and 45 percent of the women said that they were working to reduce their weight. Obviously, the 1990s saw an increase in the percentage of men working to lose weight, suggesting that the gap between the genders is closing.

We don't know all the reasons for this shift, but can surmise that it is a reflection of the increased rates of excess weight as well as progress in the recognition of the benefits of weight loss. Still, until the rates of overweight and obesity are reversed, it is clear that more men and women who are above a healthy weight or who are gaining weight as adults must decide to lose weight.

FROM A WOMAN'S VIEWPOINT
WHO'S TRYING TO LOSE WEIGHT?

There is an upside to realizing you're overweight—and it's to a woman's advantage. A study published in 2002 by researchers at the University of Florida in Gainesville, found that among women and men with the same BMI (where both have a weight classified as healthy, overweight, or obese), men are significantly more likely than women to rate their size as socially acceptable when they are overweight or obese. Since women typically identify their weight problem earlier than most men, women are more likely to do something about it sooner rather than later.

FROM A MAN'S VIEWPOINT
WHO'S TRYING TO LOSE WEIGHT?

Compared with women, men often take more time to decide to lose weight, even when they identify themselves as being overweight. A national survey of overweight men conducted in 2003 found that 23 percent of the men said they wanted to lose weight but weren't doing anything about it, 17 percent reported being on a weight-loss diet, and 13 percent had never tried to lose weight. The remaining 47 percent said they had no interest in losing weight. Unfortunately, the choice to put off losing weight placed the "no interest" guys at a higher risk of becoming even heavier and developing health problems.

It's not all bad news for men, however, because when men do decide to take the weight-loss plunge, they appear to have more realistic weight-loss goals than women. One large study of overweight male and female dieters found that women considered greater amounts of weight loss to be realistic compared with men. Being realistic offers men a weight-loss advantage because weight-loss expectations that are unachievable can be a setup for failure. When weight-loss expectations are not met, the likelihood of quitting the weight-loss effort is high—and nobody can lose weight if he or she is not even trying.

REAL-LIFE LESSON
The Great Weight-Loss Debate

Situation: My husband and I are having a debate and we'd like you to give us the answer. We will be celebrating our twenty-fifth wedding anniversary with a large party in six weeks. I say that I should be able to lose 25 pounds for the party, and my husband says that 10 to 15 pounds is more realistic. Who's right?

Strategies: Ever hear the expression "Yard by yard it may be hard, but inch by inch, it's a cinch?" In all my years with Weight Watchers, I have found that having realistic expectations about how quickly weight can be lost is key to a successful outcome. Here's what the experts agree on: After the first couple of weeks (when loss can be higher due to the loss of water), an average weight loss of 1 to 2 pounds per week is healthful, realistic, and most important, achievable. Losing weight at a greater rate—even if it can be achieved—is not a good idea because it is highly unlikely to be sustained, and the health risks of rapid weight loss rise quickly when weight loss exceeds the 2-pound-per-week mark. Although this may not be what you want to hear, it's the reality. So your husband is declared the winner of this debate. Why not set a goal of losing 10 pounds by your anniversary party? Then, if you lose 12 or 13 pounds, you will have exceeded your expectations—a lovely situation to be in.

Wrapping Things Up

Although weight has traditionally been viewed as a woman's issue, there are plenty of reasons why both men and women should be concerned about their weight.

• Currently, there are more overweight adult men than overweight adult women in this country. And although there are still more obese women than obese men, the percentage of women seems to be leveling off and that of men seems to be on the rise. Being aware that women and men view weight from quite different angles can help you and your partner in understanding and assisting each other's weight-management efforts.

- Women tend to be better than men at accurately assessing their weight status. Some women are too good, believing that they should weigh less than is healthy. On the other hand, many men might benefit from reevaluating their perceptions of a healthy weight.

- In general, women can benefit from reducing their emotional investment in their weight and working to become less concerned with others' opinions of the size of their body, while most men already do a good job of keeping their weight-related emotions in check.

- Though the gap is narrowing, more women than men are willing to make an effort to lose weight, though some women need to be more realistic about their weight-loss goals. Men are often more realistic in setting achievable goals, but many would benefit from starting a weight-loss program sooner rather than later.

Let's Talk!

Use the answers to these questions to begin to explore how you can change the lens through which you view your weight:

1. Am I overweight, and if so, by how much?

2. How does my weight make me feel? Are those feelings too strong? Not strong enough?

3. What am I doing to achieve or maintain a healthy weight?

CHAPTER 4

He's Fit, She's Thin

The Language of Weight Loss

It's 8:00 A.M. and coworkers Marcus and Jada have a breakfast meeting with colleagues from their organization's purchasing department. As they enter the conference room, they confront a buffet table jam-packed with beverages, rich pastries, giant-sized bagels, bowls of whipped cream cheese, and single-serving packages of sugary cereals. Marcus, who has recently noticed that he's put on a few pounds, pours himself a cup of coffee and takes a seat next to a male coworker who comments, "Marcus, it's hard to believe a big guy like you doesn't eat breakfast."

He says: "I'm trying to get into better shape, so I ate a light breakfast at home"

Meanwhile, Jada has maneuvered her way along the buffet table, managing to take only a carton of skim milk and half a bagel without cream cheese. She has been trying to lose weight on and off for the past year. As she takes a seat next to Marcus, a female coworker who overheard Marcus and the other man talking comments, "Are you on a diet, too?"

She says: "Since I started working here, I've gone up two dress sizes! I am dieting, and most of the stuff on the buffet table is off-limits for me."

Same meeting. Same buffet table. And yes, both Marcus and Jada are committed to losing weight. There is one major difference: Jada freely describes herself as being on a diet, while Marcus talks about getting into shape.

An interesting facet of weight management is the language that men and women use when talking about their experiences. It's especially interesting because so much scientific research has been done on excess weight and related health problems, but very few studies have looked at gender differences regarding the words and language women and men use when talking about weight loss. This is surprising, given that language is such an integral part of life, affecting our ability to understand one another and communicate effectively. Yet although academic scientists have not spent a lot of time looking at the language of weight, Weight Watchers has done extensive internal research on the topic, having talked for many years with both men and women from all over the world. The goal of this chapter is to share the results of that research and to explore the gender differences in the language of weight. Helping both women and men understand these differences can go a long way toward increasing awareness of how word choices have the potential to affect each other's weight-loss success.

Choose Your Words Carefully: How Women and Men Talk about Weight

The process of change that women and men go through to lose weight is very similar. To lose weight successfully, everyone must travel at his or her own pace through the various stages of change. Regardless of one's gender, the first step is to move from an area where weight is not even on one's radar screen to an area where one recognizes the excess weight. From there, the person prepares a plan for losing the weight, then acts on that plan, then begins to shed the excess pounds. Finally, once the behaviors that produced the weight loss are engrained in the person's daily life, the job of maintaining the new lifestyle takes hold.

While the process of changing one's behavior is the same, the words that women and men use to describe the experience are very different. A variety of market research techniques used on behalf of Weight Watchers demonstrate that women and men have their own preferred words and phrases that they use to talk about weight. In general, women talk about their weight in terms of how they look. The majority of men, on the other hand, talk about their weight using words connected to health and fitness.

The way that women and men typically describe their current weight status follows that pattern. One area in which there is agreement between the genders is in the description of obesity. Understandably, neither men nor women like to be called obese. In a quest to find more acceptable language, Weight Watchers researchers asked obese women and men to describe their weight. The women tended to describe themselves in terms that related to their appearance, covered a variety of body parts, and had negative connotations. Examples include "I look fat," "I have flabby arms," and "My rear end is huge." On the other hand, men typically answered the question using more neutral or positive phrases, such as "I've always been big" and "I'm on the heavy side." And when men did talk about their appearance, they focused almost exclusively on one body part—the stomach. They said things like "I've got a beer belly" or "I've got a big gut."

Another example of women's tendency to describe their appearance and men's tendency to talk about health and fitness is in how they describe what they want to achieve by losing weight. When researchers asked women and men to describe their weight-loss goals, women primarily used appearance-related words and phrases that have to do with looking thin. Examples of their responses include "I want to be skinnier" and "I want to wear a size 6." But descriptors relating to appearance weren't the only ones that the researchers heard from the women who wanted to lose weight. They found that women were also interested in their health, but it didn't seem to be as motivating compared to their appearance.

In the same research, the male response was very different. The researchers noted that none of the men surveyed ever used the word *thin* to describe their weight-loss goals (more on this in the next section). Instead, the men focused on health- and performance-related phrases, such as "I want to be fit" and "I want to get in shape." One man summed up the typical male response when he said, "I want to feel better. I hate being tired and sore all the time. I can't do the things that were once natural to do."

Just as there were exceptions with women in the appearance-versus-fitness divide, so, too, were there exceptions with the men. In the researchers' work with men, they heard men, particularly younger men, express concern about their appearance. Many said that they wanted to look better and fit into clothing that had become too tight or too small. One male study participant reported, "My fat pants were getting tight, and I just didn't like the way I looked."

Based on years of Weight Watchers research, we have concluded that the way in which women and men talk to each other appears to have a profound impact on their weight-loss efforts. Many of the words that women and men tend to use can also have either a positive or a negative effect on the emotional reactions of someone of the opposite gender, and that effect can make a difference to the other's weight-loss success.

FROM A WOMAN'S VIEWPOINT
CHOOSE YOUR WORDS CAREFULLY: HOW WOMEN
AND MEN TALK ABOUT WEIGHT

Most men want to encourage the women in their lives when it comes to losing weight. But when women talk about their experience, they tend to use words and concepts that are alien to most men's weight-loss vocabulary. For example, women often talk about their feelings of being sabotaged in their weight-loss efforts. In a study that looked at this notion, the idea of sabotage was not a concept that the average man could relate to when talking about weight loss. In the same research, women were also much more likely to describe feelings of disgust or remorse after an episode of overeating. Again, the men had a hard time relating to those emotionally charged descriptions. So what happens? Women may feel that their partners are not listening or don't care when they talk about the weight-loss issues they are dealing with. To overcome that barrier, women need to keep the word differences in mind when they talk about their weight with the men in their lives. A lack of understanding should not be automatically equated with a lack of caring. Finding a common language with which to express the feelings can make all the difference.

FROM A MAN'S VIEWPOINT
CHOOSE YOUR WORDS CAREFULLY: HOW WOMEN
AND MEN TALK ABOUT WEIGHT

Men often use sports terminology when talking about their weight, such as "I'm as big as a linebacker" or "I've got a wrestler's body—thick and stocky." Men also tend to see those self-assessments as factual, even complimentary. Weight Watchers research has found that male-dominated descriptions often go back to childhood, when boys played sports and were encouraged to be "muscular" or "big" or "fast" or "strong."

Even though many women also played sports when they were young, the words that are complimentary to guys do not necessarily cross the gender divide. In fact, girls who played sports and were described as big, muscular, or big-boned did not generally take the words as compliments. For many women those words translate as "fat." So when guys are talking with women about weight, they need to leave the locker-room language behind and be sensitive to the fact that most women do not appreciate being called "a big woman" or having someone notice that they have "really bulked up" since they began working out. Men would be much better off using language that compliments a woman's appearance, like "nice curves" or "you look so much more toned since you began working out."

REAL-LIFE LESSON
Weight Loss—A Touchy Subject

Situation: I'm a thirty-year-old guy who recently achieved a healthy weight, having lost about 25 pounds. I stopped playing sports in high school, and in college I started noticing that my weight was creeping up. I put on more weight in my twenties. So I started going to the gym and watching what I ate, and the weight came off. But now I'm concerned about my younger sister. She just started a new job and she is the heaviest I've ever seen her. I want to talk with her about her weight, but she's very sensitive about it. Any thoughts on how to bring up the subject? I really want to help her.

Strategies: You are a terrific brother! A fundamental difference between men and women is that most men do not appreciate unsolicited support, while women often thrive on it. I suggest that you speak with your sister about how much your weight-loss success has improved your life—how it has given you more energy, how you feel better about yourself and can even get into a suit from your college years. Let your sister know that you'd like to share the benefits of your success with her if she's interested. That doesn't mean telling her what you think she needs to do to fix her problem, but rather telling her that you want to be there to support her. Why not invite her to your gym, have her over to your place for a light meal, or ask her to take a Sunday-morning hike with you? When it comes to weight loss, success is contagious. Let your sister catch your success and then encourage her as she finds her way.

Lost in Translation

When it comes to discussing weight, it's almost as if women and men are speaking different languages. Not only do they use different words to describe the same weight-loss experiences, but they also often use the same word to convey a completely different meaning. Weight Watchers has been able to identify key words that, when used inappropriately by the opposite sex, can result in miscommunication and bad feelings. Here's a snapshot of what the research has decoded so far. Think of it as a gender-sensitive weight-loss dictionary to help decipher the meaning of particular words.

big   *adj.:* of great size, large, bulky

Woman's translation: If you want to insult a woman, just call her "big." Overweight women would rather be referred to as full-figured, curvy, or well-endowed.

Man's translation: Men generally don't take offense at being called "big." In fact, many view it as a compliment; it makes them sound large, strong, and in charge.

challenge   *n.:* a calling into question, a call to a duel, anything that demands special effort

Woman's translation: When talking about weight loss, the word *challenge* resonates negatively with women. A challenge sounds hard, difficult, something they would like to avoid. Using the word *challenge* with women can make them feel overwhelmed. Women often prefer to use the word *journey* to describe their weight-loss efforts.

Man's translation: Men react positively to the word *challenge* in terms of describing how best to lose weight—it is part of their sports vocabulary. To guys, a challenge appeals to their sense of competition and can even motivate them to lose weight.

choice *n.:* a selection, the right or power to choose, the best part, an alternative or variety from which to choose

Woman's translation: Since women tend to be detail-oriented when it comes to losing weight (see chapter 8), they prefer to have several options in going about it. To a woman the word *choice* is viewed positively and means that she will have a wide variety of options from which she can choose.

Man's translation: Men, on the other hand, are much more oriented to the bottom line in the way they plan to lose weight (see chapter 8). When first attempting to shed excess pounds, they are not looking for a lot of choices. Most guys prefer to keep their choices simple—for example, they want a list of "eat" foods and "don't eat" foods. As they progress, most men look for substitutions for their favorite foods rather than more choices.

crave *v.t.:* to long for eagerly; to beg for earnestly

Woman's translation: Chocolate. Ice cream. No matter where a woman is in the course of life—for example, pregnant, experiencing PMS, or menopausal—she is likely to get cravings for certain foods. Cravings are those intense feelings of "I've got to have it now" or "I'm in the mood for ——." Cravings often prompt women to overeat. Consequently, cravings are often viewed negatively by women who are in weight-loss mode.

Man's translation: Intellectually, men know what cravings are, but they often view them as a woman thing. When it comes to losing weight, men don't typically experience cravings in the same way that women do. They are more likely to simply eat the food that they want, enjoy the food, not feel particularly guilty when they have it, then get on with their weight-loss efforts. Men really don't have a comparable word for *craving* because they have a hard time relating to the concept.

diet *n.:* what a person usually eats or drinks; a special or limited selection of foods and beverages chosen or prescribed to bring about weight loss

Woman's translation: Women love to use the word *diet* or its many variations and often identify with the concept: "I am on a diet," or "I am dieting," or "I am a dieter." In fact, women often use the word *diet* when describing any weight-loss regimen, even a comprehensive approach that includes exercise, thinking skills, and a supportive environment.

Man's translation: Although men under the age of forty-five are starting to use the word *diet,* many men still view dieting as a female phenomenon and a negative one at that. Rather than diet, men "change their lifestyle" (which is often used as a synonym for eating differently) and "get in shape."

exercise *n.:* performance or activity for developing the body or mind

Woman's translation: Exercise is something that athletes do. Women prefer to engage in physical activity; they work out, take aerobics classes, do yoga, and use hand weights.

Man's translation: Exercise is a macho word; men enjoy exercising and consider it a fundamental way to lose their guts and get in shape. Men run, play sports, hit the gym, and pump iron.

support *v.t.:* to carry the weight of; to hold up; to encourage or help; to bear or endure

Woman's translation: Most women seek a great deal of emotional and psychological *support* when losing weight. To a woman, *support* means "help and encouragement from other people"—friends, coworkers, family members, and loved ones such as a husband or boyfriend. Women often feel sabotaged when they don't get support from others.

Man's translation: Men also use the word *support* when talking about weight loss, but they are referring more to technical and physical support than to emotional support. From the male perspective, support is being advised about what to order from a menu or which foods to purchase at the supermarket. Certainly, many men turn to their wives or other women for help with those types of choices. But when the typical man talks about support, he means assistance from someone whose expertise on the topic exceeds his own.

thin   *adj.:* lean, slender, skinny

Woman's translation: In our thin-obsessed culture, most women see being described as thin as the ultimate compliment. Indeed, *thin* is a very popular word among women describing how they would like to look. And when a woman has lost weight, it's a major compliment to say that she looks thin.

Man's translation: For many men, *thin* is a synonym for *unhealthy*; it implies a weak and wimpy man. It would be insulting to say to a man, "You look so thin!" Instead, men prefer being called "fit" or "less heavy" or "in better shape."

FROM A WOMAN'S VIEWPOINT
LOST IN TRANSLATION

When it comes to losing weight, many women are notorious for making black-and-white statements like "I'll never eat chocolate again!" or "I'm on a diet, so no more desserts." The reality is that it won't be long before they're nibbling on a bite-size candy bar or ordering a small slice of cheesecake when eating out. What's going on? Weight Watchers research has found that compared with men, women often take poetic license, making sweeping statements to describe their weight-loss efforts. What women mean is that they are going to eat some foods in smaller portions or less frequently but not necessarily avoid them forever. The "never-again" declarations can be frustrating for men, who are inclined to take such language literally. The problem with this particular miscommunication is that it can lead a man to believe that his wife, daughter, or female friend is not serious about losing weight, so he may provide less support and encouragement than he might otherwise.

FROM A MAN'S VIEWPOINT
LOST IN TRANSLATION

Men tend to be literal-minded and goal-oriented, especially when it comes to losing weight. If the meal plan says he can't have wine, he won't have wine. If the meal plan says he can eat steak and eggs, then he will eat steak and eggs. While this male logic may seem simplistic, researchers believe that it helps men set and accomplish their weight-loss goals—many of which are not based on the number on the bathroom scale. What are some of men's weight-loss goals? A couple of examples from some male subscribers to Weight Watchers Online are "I need to get down to my riding weight so that I fit into my race leathers comfortably" and "I want to get into the weight range that will get me the lowest rates for life insurance."

A word of advice to women who want to help their overweight men lose weight: there's no need to ask a lot of questions. Guys are more straightforward—if they set a weight-loss goal, chances are they will follow through with it.

REAL-LIFE LESSON
I Need To Lose Weight and I Need Your Support

Situation: I've been losing weight, and everyone seems to have noticed—my boss, the members of my church group—everyone except my fiancé. He says that I look great and he doesn't care what size I am. But I have type 2 diabetes and my doctor told me I need to lose weight. How can I talk to him so that he can understand how important losing weight is to me?

Strategies: The best approach is for you to have a straightforward conversation with your fiancé that puts the importance of your weight loss into a context that he can relate to and then provide him with specific things that he can do to support your efforts. For example, you could say that you are working with your doctor to get your diabetes under control (which will be important if the two of you are planning to have children), that weight loss is key to that goal, and that you'd appreciate his asking about the results of your bloodwork after your visits to the doctor. What is unlikely to work is asking him to notice and compliment you when you've lost a few pounds or to expect a weight-related compliment when asking a vague question like "How do I look?" From what you say, that is not a context he can relate to, so give him a break on this and rely on your church group and coworkers to support you on that front.

The Weight-Loss Gender Evolution

Over the past couple of decades, our society has experienced some profound gender-role shifts in a variety of areas, including education, employment, and family life. In the realm of family life, for example, men have become more involved in childrearing. Remember the traditional fathers, who never changed a baby's diaper (and if they did, they would never admit it) because that was considered a woman's job? Well, those men are gone! In the 1980s and 1990s dads began not only changing diapers but enjoying it. Now, in the twenty-first century, we're seeing a second generation of diaper-changing dads, many of them carrying masculine-looking diaper bags.

What does changing diapers have to do with losing weight? Just as men traditionally viewed childrearing as women's work, men have

Ed Schmitt and his daughter Jennifer
NEW YORK

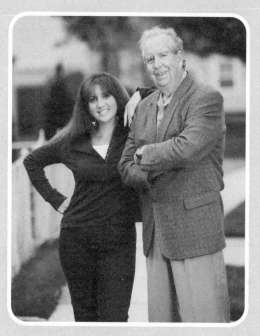

Ed is fifty-seven years old and has been married to his wife, Jo, for thirty-seven years. They have four grown children, Jennifer, Kristopher, Danille, and Brett. Ed is the chief financial officer for an electronics firm; Jennifer, his thirty-four-year-old daughter, works in the corporate office of a merchandising company. She lives at home with her parents and sometimes finds herself commuting up to four hours a day.

Although Ed's wife has never had a weight problem, Ed has been overweight for years but for the most part was unaware of it. He says, "I never thought of myself as fat; I just considered myself big—I'm six feet three inches tall and the least I can remember weighing is two hundred fifteen pounds—when I was twenty-one years old!" He adds, "I assumed that my incremental weight gains over the years were part of growing older." In 2005, on a visit to his doctor, Ed discovered that his weight had crept up to 285 pounds. He describes his condition: "My blood pressure was out of whack, I had diabetes, and my doctor told me that if I wanted to be around for the long term, I'd better think seriously about losing weight." Ed said initially he felt down. He says, "I thought it was too late for me to change." But after the birth of his first grandchild, Tyler, he was motivated to make some long-needed changes. He had heard that Weight Watchers was the most practical and realistic way to lose weight. He says, "In my mind I understood that I wasn't starting a diet; I was making a lifestyle change."

After joining Weight Watchers, Ed soon realized that his weight gain had been a result of what he ate during the day when he was away from home. He explains, "My wife cooks only healthy foods. I was eating all kinds of junk at work, and when I came home, I was a couch potato." After a year, Ed had lost 65.2 pounds; he reached his weight goal and is now a Weight Watchers Lifetime member. Ed vows that he'll never be heavy again. He says, "I don't even need an alarm clock. At six A.M., I'm up and walking three miles at least five mornings a week. I'm also eating breakfast, which I never used to do."

Although Ed was concerned about Jennifer's weight, he never said a word to her about it. After her thirty-fourth birthday, she decided to fix the things in her life that she felt were broken and decided that losing weight and feeling better about her appearance were great places to start. She says, "After my dad had been going to Weight Watchers for just ten weeks, I was totally impressed with his weight-loss success. I figured if it worked for Dad, it could work for me." Jennifer asked her dad about joining, and they agreed to help each other out. Every Wednesday they attend a meeting together. She says, "I love going to meetings with my dad. It's a special time for both of us. And my supervisors at work have been so supportive. They know how important losing weight is to me and they have allowed me to make up the time I take off so that I can attend the meetings with my dad."

Jennifer started Weight Watchers at 226 pounds and has lost sixty-seven pounds so far. She says, "I've gone from a size eighteen dress size to a ten or twelve, and it just feels terrific to buy clothes and feel great wearing them." One thing that Jennifer does that's different from what her dad does involves exercise. She explains, "I don't have time with my long commute, so I am very careful about what and how much I eat. I know exercise is important, but for now I'm focusing on my eating."

Jennifer says that without her dad's support and encouragement, she's not sure she would have been successful. Ed agrees. He says, "Jen and I are a team. We keep each other honest and motivated."

viewed weight loss as a female phenomenon, and a negative one at that. But men's views appear to be changing: they are more likely to decide to lose weight and are acknowledging that they are following a specific weight-loss method to accomplish it.

Women's views are changing, too. Women have taken notice of men's success at weight loss and are beginning to seek their advice and ask about their experiences.

But why are more men making the commitment to lose weight? There are no doubt several reasons, including the undeniable fact that there are now more overweight and obese men than ever before. But Weight Watchers research also suggests that when it comes to men, age matters. Based on a large study conducted in 2006, Weight Watchers discovered that while men over the age of forty-five said that their primary reason for losing weight was health-related, for men under the age of forty-five the reason cited most often was to look better and get in shape.

Age also seems to play a role in the method chosen to lose weight. Although men tend to rely more on exercise than women, the study found that both younger and older men are also changing their eating behaviors. And although men in both age groups are changing those behaviors, the age groups differ in the changes they are making. Older men, particularly those with quite a bit of weight to lose, said that they had found limited success by reducing their overall food intake—often they reduce or eliminate carbohydrate-rich foods, eliminate alcohol, and consume meal-replacement shakes. Younger men said that they are using those eating strategies as well, but they are also exercising more than the older guys. In fact, it was not uncommon for men under the age of forty-five to say that they exercise three or more times a week and spend four or more hours doing it.

So why are guys getting on the weight-loss bandwagon and going public with their efforts? In a phrase, *they need to*. Older guys are getting the news from their doctors that those years of gaining weight are catching up with them. Men tend to be natural problem-solvers, and there's nothing to motivate a guy to lose weight like the diagnosis of a life-shortening disease. And for the younger guys, the media may be a key. Just as women have been bombarded for decades with images of superthin women, men are now getting similar treatment. Marketers are targeting men with ads featuring young, athletic male models with six-pack abs and a percentage of body fat in the low single digits. Those Adonis-like male bodies have undoubtedly persuaded some men, particularly the younger ones, to take action.

Whether it is health or appearance that motivates the decision to lose weight, the good news for both genders is that the opportunity to have constructive conversations about weight has never been greater. Both women and men recognize the importance of losing weight. If women and men can learn to understand and adapt to their unique ways of talking about weight, they can help each other learn the strategies that work and encourage each other's weight-loss progress.

FROM A WOMAN'S VIEWPOINT
THE WEIGHT-LOSS GENDER EVOLUTION

If a woman really wants to encourage that special man in her life to lose some weight, it may help to discuss the issue like a man. Men love challenges. Weight Watchers research in Australia suggests that women may be more effective if they use language that appeals to a man's sense of competition and fitness. For example, instead of saying, "Honey, you'd look better if you lost some weight," a more effective tactic may be to appeal to the man's sense of competition by saying something like "I bet you couldn't lose ten pounds over the next six weeks." Chances are that men will respond to that approach and take on the challenge.

FROM A MAN'S VIEWPOINT
THE WEIGHT-LOSS GENDER EVOLUTION

A woman's weight is a subject most men would rather not bring up, but it shouldn't be avoided. A man can provide a woman with invaluable encouragement if he understands how to listen to the meaning behind her words and then respond in a supportive way. Since women tend to be highly focused on their appearance, men can be actively supportive by providing positive feedback, such as "You've lost some weight, and you look terrific!" or "I am so proud of how you are taking care of yourself." And since some women have unrealistic expectations about how much they should weigh, men can help validate a more realistic weight and size with statements such as "Please don't lose too much weight" or "You've reached a BMI of twenty-five—that's terrific!"

REAL-LIFE LESSON
Fit or Fat?

Situation: My uncle is overweight, but he insists that he's in good shape because he lifts weights and jogs on the treadmill several times a week. I told him he needs to lose weight, but he disagrees and says he is fit. As his only niece, how can I help him understand that I am concerned about his health? My dad, his brother, was also overweight, and he died last year of a heart attack.

Strategies: The concept of "fit or fat" and its cousins "fit and fat" and "not fit and not fat" are topics of much scientific debate. Experts agree, however, that to be fit and not fat is best. I'd suggest a two-tactic approach in reaching your uncle. First, there is information on this topic at the Science Center at WeightWatchers.com (www .WeightWatchers.com/science). Since most guys like expert information from a reliable source, I suggest that you either print out the articles for him or use the e-mail feature at the site to get the information into his hands. That tactic should take the conversation from "you say, he says" to one based on the facts. Second, I suggest that you appeal to the things you already know are important to him: being fit and in shape. Rather than focus on your concern that he's going to carry on the family tradition of having a heart attack, point out what *better* shape he'll be in and how he can become even *fitter* by adding a food plan to his already admirable exercise regimen. I am confident that if he takes the first step, the results he sees will motivate him to strive to be both fit and trim.

Wrapping Things Up

Weight is a hot conversation topic, but unfortunately many women and men have trouble discussing it with each other. Part of the reason is miscommunication: women and men seem to speak different weight-loss languages.

- Women and men use different words to describe their weight and their weight-loss efforts. Women tend to use colorful words such as *fat* and *flabby*, words that focus on appearance and often paint an unflattering picture; men often use sports terminology, such as *big* and *large,* and focus on health and/or performance. Men are also more likely than women to express their weight and weight-loss efforts in more positive terms.

- Even when men and women use the same words, the words can have very different or even opposite meanings. Women view *thin* as a compliment, while men tend to view it as an insult, translating it as "weak" or "wimpy."

- The gender-based world of weight loss is evolving—and it's to both women's and men's benefit. Men are more likely to commit themselves to weight loss and are willing to discuss their experience more publicly. As a result, women are beginning to seek out men for weight-related advice.

Let's Talk!

Not sure which language you're speaking when you're having a weight-related conversation? Here are some questions that can help stimulate conversation between women and men and put them on the same page:

1. What words would you use to describe your desirable weight?

2. Are there any particular words that you find offensive when used to describe your weight or what you're doing to lose weight?

3. How would you feel about working as a couple to lose weight?

CHAPTER 5

Why Guys Lose Weight Faster

Brad and Irene are sitting by a roaring fire on New Year's Eve, waiting for their twin teenage sons to return home safely. At the stroke of midnight, they propose a toast to celebrate their New Year's resolutions: Brad's vow to get in shape and Irene's commitment to losing weight. Brad recently noticed that he's put on a few pounds and feels soft around the middle, and he has made the resolution to exercise more. Irene put on weight when she was pregnant with the twins. Despite the fact that their kids are now in their teens, she has never successfully shed the baby weight. For the New Year she has made a commitment to cook family meals and stop eating late at night, a habit she developed when the twins started driving and she began waiting up for them.

After a few weeks, they have both made progress; Brad has lost 6 pounds and Irene has lost 3 pounds. Brad is not surprised that he has had some success: he says, "I think working out every day on my lunch break has helped me get back into shape."

A few weeks later, Brad has continued to lose twice as much weight as Irene. Frustrated and ready to toss the bathroom scale out the window, she says, "It's not fair! Men lose weight so much faster than women. I'm eating better and snacking less but my body refuses to lose weight more quickly!"

Couples like Irene and Brian who have decided to lose weight at the same time have probably noticed that the man usually loses more weight and at a faster pace than the woman. What's going on? The truth is that men do have a physical edge over women in terms of weight loss—their body composition enables them to lose more weight than a woman of the same weight. But women have an edge over men in other critical areas of weight management: women tend to be more attentive to what's going on with their weight and are better able to make the connection between food and emotions.

This chapter examines why men and women not only talk about the issue of excess weight differently but why they experience it differently as well.

Where Did the Weight Come From?

There is no denying that both women and men gain weight as the years pass. The average weight gain for adult men is 1.7 pounds per year and for women, 1.4 pounds. More than half say that they've gained at least 20 pounds since reaching adulthood. And the trend seems to be worsening. Among adults between the ages of eighteen and thirty-four, the average weight gain per year is 2.7 pounds for men and 2.2 pounds for women.

In a survey of overweight men and women conducted for Weight Watchers, women reported actively working at weight management for a longer period of time than their male counterparts. While part of that difference can undoubtedly be attributed to women's earlier awareness of the excess weight and a quicker decision to take action, the age at which a substantial amount of weight was gained also seems to have played a role. In the survey, 56 percent of the women reported becoming overweight in their twenties. Only 43 percent of the men in the survey said that their twenties was their decade of substantial weight gain. The women in the survey also reported gaining their weight in a shorter period of time compared with the men.

When it comes to life events that trigger a substantial weight gain, the sexes are both similar and different. In another Weight Watchers study, overweight men and women were asked to describe life events that lead to weight gain. In equal numbers, the women and the men linked quitting smoking, going to college, starting a new job, getting married, and getting divorced to weight gain. Men were much more likely than women to associate a gain in weight with a slowdown (or stop) in exercise, as well as with an illness or injury. Three times more women than men, however, linked the death of a family member to a weight gain. Although it is not surprising that 46 percent of women cited having children as a life event that led to weight gain, it may be surprising to note that 6 percent of men did, too. Finally, menopause was cited as a major time of weight gain for women.

FROM A WOMAN'S VIEWPOINT
WHERE DID THE WEIGHT COME FROM?

Most women know that having a baby (or two or three or more) puts her in a weight-precarious situation. Women at a healthy weight are encouraged to gain about 25 pounds over the course of a pregnancy. Those who go into a pregnancy overweight are encouraged to gain a bit less, 15 to 25 pounds. While gaining the weight usually isn't diffi-cult for most women (and exceeding the recommended weight gain is not uncommon), taking off the excess weight once the baby is born can be a challenge. It's hard for some women even to remember what they looked like or felt like before getting pregnant. This is even truer if there are multiple babies over a few years, in which case the likelihood of returning to the pre-baby weight and shape doesn't occur before a new one is on the way. In addition, the demands of the new baby often leave moms with little time or energy to put effort into their daily eating and exercise routines. Not surprisingly, many overweight women report that having a baby or babies and not taking off all the extra weight they gained while pregnant is one of the key factors leading to an ongoing battle with their weight.

After the baby years, women eventually face another challenge that for many is weight-related: menopause. While the typical weight gain at this time of life is 5 to 7 pounds, larger gains are not uncommon. In addition, the hormonal changes that come with menopause cause a change in body shape, with weight accumulating around the waist rather than on the hips and thighs. All of those changes can take a toll on a woman's good humor, leading to negative feelings and overeating in response. (See chapter 3 for more on emotions and weight.) A study by the University of Pennsylvania School of Medicine found that middle-aged women who reported high levels of symptoms indicative of depression and anxiety were more likely to experience greater amounts of weight gain.

FROM A MAN'S VIEWPOINT
WHERE DID THE WEIGHT COME FROM?

Although some men, particularly athletes, might be asked to gain weight to enhance their physical performance, men typically do not find themselves in situations where there is a biological vulnerability to gaining weight. Hence, the tendency is that weight gain in men is a slower process. Forty-one percent of the men participating in a survey of Weight Watchers Online subscribers reported that they gained their weight slowly.

The landscape of weight gain for men appears to be shifting, however, and the factor that separates the men from the boys is age. For guys who are part of or older than the baby boom generation, a weight gain related to smoking cessation is much more likely than it is for younger men. Conversely, men in their twenties and thirties are significantly more likely than their elders to gain weight as a result of getting married, going away to college, starting a new job, and having children. When it comes to times in the life cycle when men gain weight, it appears that younger men have more in common with women than do older men. While there may be many reasons for that, such as fewer differences in the way gender roles are now defined by society, the news is not good for today's young men insofar as weight is concerned. With the rates of overweight and obesity among men on the rise, it's not good that they are putting on the pounds at a younger age than their fathers did.

REAL-LIFE LESSON
Preventing Postpartum Pounds

Situation: I'm twenty-nine and had a baby six months ago. I don't know what's wrong with me: I just can't seem to get rid of the extra pounds. I've just joined Weight Watchers but I'm not losing weight at the pace that I could when I was younger. I am frustrated because I can't fit into any of my prepregnancy clothes. Any suggestions?

Strategies: First and most important, you need to be patient. It's truly sad that so many Hollywood celebrity moms have created a belief that a woman can return to her pre-baby weight and shape within days or weeks of giving birth. Those woman often have full-time trainers and chefs to help them shed their weight. They also have a great deal of motivation because their ability to earn a living often depends on their being able to take drastic steps to get weight off. In other words, they do not live average lives—but the rest of us do. It's a rare woman who returns to her prepregnancy weight without more time and effort than it's taken to lose weight in the past. Most new mothers are overwhelmed by so many changes—breastfeeding, hormonal peaks and valleys, sleep deprivation—all of which can make it difficult to adhere strictly to a weight-loss plan.

Congratulations for joining Weight Watchers; it will help you to structure both your eating and your exercising in a way that is healthful and feasible. Attending a weekly meeting may be just what you need to stay motivated and accountable to your weight-loss effort. You'll be losing weight now at a recommended pace, and that will enhance your health and ensure a strong body, especially in the event of another child.

One strategy that may be helpful is weaving a weight-loss schedule into the baby's schedule. One tactic is preparing your meals during nap times and sticking them in the refrigerator. Taking long walks with the stroller to get in some exercise is another. Most important, finding a way to attend the weekly meeting is a must. Many Weight Watchers locations have meetings that you can attend with your young ones so that finding a babysitter isn't necessary. Alternatively, attending a meeting during your lunch hour (assuming you've returned to work) or leaving Dad in charge for an evening meeting may work best. If attending a meeting simply isn't possible, subscribing to Weight Watchers Online is a good option. Regardless of your choice, the message boards on WeightWatchers.com can be a terrific source of encouragement and inspiration. Feeling supported is critical to weight-loss success—and that's especially true for new moms.

Why Men and Women Think They Gain and How They Think They Lose

When it comes to what people think is responsible for weight gain, there is a clear divide between the sexes. In general, women are more likely to accept personal responsibility for a weight gain than men, acknowledging that the choices that they've made to eat too much food and not get enough exercise are the roots of their weight status. Unfortunately, some women go too far in accepting responsibility for their weight gain, turning it into an exercise in self-blame and guilt. Although taking responsibility and learning from past behaviors are important to making a positive change, dwelling on past errors and wishing they hadn't happened is not helpful when it comes to achieving lasting weight loss.

Compared with women, men are less likely to accept personal responsibility for their weight status. Research conducted for Weight Watchers found that men are more likely to believe that they are overweight because of hereditary reasons or on account of the way they ate growing up. Men are more likely than women to view gaining weight as something that just "happened" and over which they had little control. But once men decide that the excess weight is a problem that they want to fix, they are very willing to accept responsibility for what needs to be done and take action.

Another area in which the genders tend to differ in their beliefs is choosing the best approach to losing weight. Many guys put their faith in exercise, and there are logical reasons for that. First, men are more likely than women to believe that a reduction in or lack of exercise was at the root of their weight gain, so it makes sense to them that revving up that aspect of their daily life would be the solution for reversing the problem. Confidence may play a role as well. Because many guys have more confidence in their ability to exercise than in their ability to make wise food choices, they often turn to physical activity to lose weight, leaving out of the mix the concept of reducing their intake of calories from food.

Women take a different approach. Although most women recognize that exercise is an important factor in the weight equation, they are less likely to use it as a primary weight-loss method, relying instead on reducing calories from food. And just like guys, confidence may play a role in the decision. Women's confidence when it comes to exercise lags behind that of most men. Women do tend to be confident, however, in their knowledge of food and how it can be used in the weight-loss process.

FROM A WOMAN'S VIEWPOINT
WHY MEN AND WOMEN THINK THEY GAIN
AND HOW THEY THINK THEY LOSE

Feeling down? Grab some ice cream. Job too stressful? Polish off some chocolate chip cookies. Many women attribute their excess weight to eating when their emotional state is in the negative zone—when they are feeling sad, stressed, or tired. Research conducted for Weight Watchers found that women are much more likely than men to attribute their weight gain to negative emotional factors. Making the connection between negative feelings and overeating, then having a list of nonfood "makes-me-feel-better" things to do when the blues strike can be one of the best tactics in a weight-loss bag of tricks.

FROM A MAN'S VIEWPOINT
WHY MEN AND WOMEN THINK THEY GAIN
AND HOW THEY THINK THEY LOSE

Men also tend to be emotional eaters—they just don't know it. While women frequently overeat when they are feeling down, men are most vulnerable to overeating when they experience the positive emotions of happiness and joy. Whether they're at a party, ball game, sports bar, or family picnic, men usually find themselves eating, drinking, and enjoying the food when they're having fun. A study sponsored by Weight Watchers found that 44 percent of overweight men said that they overeat when they're having a good time, not when they are stressed, depressed, or tense. Maintaining awareness of the amount and type of food they're eating during the fun times can be a real asset in most men's weight-loss efforts.

REAL-LIFE LESSON

Getting Guys to Balance Eating and Exercise

Situation: My husband knows that he needs to lose weight but he thinks that all he has to do is exercise and the pounds will disappear. I told him that he needs to change his eating habits, too, but he says that's not necessary. Is there anything I can do to help him see the light?

Strategies: You are wise to encourage your husband to think in terms of both eating and exercising. Exercising is a great thing, but exercising alone will not get your husband to the place he wants to be. He needs to limit his intake of calories if he wants to have a substantial weight loss.

Why not have your husband do some how-much-exercise-does-it-take math—it might help him change his mind. Here are the facts: A person needs to exercise enough to burn about 5½ calories per pound of body weight per day in order to *maintain* his or her body weight. For a man weighing 200 pounds, that means burning about 1,100 calories, which is roughly equivalent to walking 11 miles, shooting hoops for 2½ to 3 hours, or hitting balls at the driving range for 4 hours. To go beyond maintaining and lose 1 pound of fat solely through exercise, a person needs to burn an additional 3,500 calories. That means that the same 200-pound man would need to walk or run an additional 5 to 10 miles per day to lose 1 to 2 pounds per week! The bottom line: Although it is theoretically possible to lose weight through exercise alone, the amount of daily exercise that it takes is not realistic for most people.

Brian and Brandi Feireisel
KENTUCKY

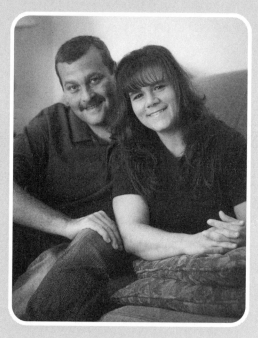

At the age of nineteen, Brandi married Brian, and they've been together for fifteen years. They have two children, Hanna, who is thirteen, and Branden, who is eight. Brian and Brandi work at the same plant, which is owned by a large automotive company. Brian works days and Brandi works the night shift; that way they both help take care of the kids.

Brandi was not overweight as a child; her weight problems started after she had her children. She reports, "I gained one hundred pounds with my daughter but lost only thirty. Then I gained seventy pounds with my son and lost very little. I struggled with my weight for twelve years and became very depressed. I was embarrassed to be with friends and family. I ran from cameras and hated looking at myself in the mirror." In high school, Brandi had been involved with many clubs and was even on the homecoming court. After she gained so much weight, people said hurtful things to her, commenting on how pretty she "used to be."

Over the years, Brandi tried fad diets and failed at all of them. That made her depression worse. When she heard some friends at work talking about Weight Watchers, she decided to join. "Weight Watchers works!" she says. "It changed my life. My depression is gone, and I've lost about seventy-three pounds. My dress size has gone from a 22–24 to a 9–10, and I just bought my first bikini!"

Her 6-foot-2-inch husband, Brian, has always been a big guy. "I've never paid much attention to my weight—I never exercised or dieted," says Brian. Over the years he gained weight, but he's not sure why, as he really never changed anything he was doing. He also takes medication for high blood pressure. "My dad was big in the middle like me and had high blood pressure, so I guess I take after him." He says that he knew he could stand to lose a few pounds but he never really thought about it much.

After Brandi joined Weight Watchers, the whole family started eating better, and not only did Brandi lose weight, but Brian lost 25 pounds as well. He says, "I feel better, and my doctor just cut my blood pressure medicine in half." Brandi does most of the shopping and Brian does the cooking. He explains, "She buys healthier foods like fruits and vegetables, and I love to catch bluegill with my son. I don't fry anymore; we bake our fish. And when I make green beans, I don't use bacon fat anymore. Now I use a seasoning that Brandi buys, and we actually like it better."

Brian feels that Brandi's weight loss has been the best thing that could have happened to the family. "Brandi looks great and feels better—her depression is totally gone," says Brian. Brandi feels that the key to her success has been her husband, the support from her fellow Weight Watchers members (she's never missed a meeting!), and the structure of her Weight Watchers food plan. According to Brandi, "I'm never hungry anymore and my food plan lets me go to a birthday party and eat the cake, too!"

How Women and Men *Really* Lose Weight

Do men really lose weight faster then women, or does it just seem that they do? The truth is that men have two key weight-loss advantages over women. One involves their body composition, which enables them to burn calories at a faster rate than women. The second is the fact that men tend to be more active than their female counterparts. The combined effect—more calories burned at rest and more calories burned in activity—translates into faster weight loss for guys.

Why are men's metabolisms faster? Men are designed by nature to have higher amounts of lean body mass, or muscle, than women. Lean body mass is the key factor that determines the rate of one's metabolism, the body's calorie-burning system. Since men have more muscle, their metabolisms are higher, and they burn more calories even when they're resting. The result is quicker weight loss. How much faster are men's metabolisms than women's? Research has shown that on average the metabolism of a man is 5 to 10 percent higher than that of a woman of the same weight and height. And because men tend to be taller and heavier than women, the male advantage on the calorie front is even greater.

Another reason men often lose weight faster then women is that they tend to be more physically active. A study reported in the *American Journal of Physiology* found that women burn an average of 16 percent fewer daily calories than men. The researchers looked into that difference, finding that the women's resting metabolic rate was 6 percent lower than that of men (i.e., a slower metabolism) and that the calories burned in physical activity were 37 percent lower than that of men. In other words, the women were simply not moving as much and so were burning fewer calories.

FROM A WOMAN'S VIEWPOINT
HOW WOMEN AND MEN *REALLY* LOSE WEIGHT

Although it may not seem fair that the differences between men's bodies and women's bodies naturally enable men to burn more calories than women, if women want to achieve better weight-loss results, it's to their advantage to pick up their exercise pace so that they can burn more calories. Since losing 1 pound of fat requires burning about 3,500 calories, anything that's done to burn those calories counts. Whether it's consuming fewer calories so that the body has to break down some of its fat to meet its basic needs or burning the calories directly by exercising (or, ideally, a combination of the two), a calorie is a calorie, and being more active can boost weight loss.

FROM A MAN'S VIEWPOINT
HOW WOMEN AND MEN *REALLY* LOSE WEIGHT

Whereas men do have a calorie-burning advantage over women, they still have to trim the calories from food in order to lose a meaningful amount of weight. Need proof? In a 3-month study, fifty-three obese men were assigned to one of four regimens: following a reduced-calorie diet, following a diet plus an exercise routine, following an exercise routine alone, and doing nothing to lose weight. Men in both the groups that included the reduced-calorie diet lost on average 17.6 pounds; those in the groups that relied solely on exercise or did nothing lost nothing. So although the weight loss was found only in the guys who trimmed calories from food, there was an advantage to the diet-plus-exercise group. The men in that group lost an average of 2.8 pounds more body fat.

REAL-LIFE LESSON
Working Out the Exercise Options

Situation: My wife is constantly on a diet. She loses some weight but then she gains most of it back. I've told her she really needs to get into a vigorous exercise routine, but she says she doesn't like that idea because she doesn't like to drip with sweat. Whenever she tries to up the exercise, she keeps it up for only about two weeks and then quits. Is there any exercise program that can help women lose weight?

Strategies: Exercise is important for both women and men. Exercise burns calories, firms and tones muscles, prevents age-related bone loss, and improves mood. People who exercise regularly also maintain their weight loss more successfully. But—and this is a big but—the truth is that all activity burns calories and there is no rule that says a person has to soak through workout clothes for exercise to contribute to weight loss. In fact, most weight-loss experts agree that activities that are done at a moderate level of intensity (like walking briskly, doing yard work, playing doubles tennis, swimming, and playing a round of golf without using a cart) are preferred for weight loss because one can do them for relatively long periods of time without quitting from exhaustion. So rather than encouraging your wife to follow a high-intensity exercise regimen, why not help her find activities that she enjoys and will feel good about doing? Better yet, find moderate-intensity activities you can do together. You might be surprised by how much fun you'll both have!

Check out the charts and compare the differences between men and women with regard to their muscle, fat, and bone distributions. Keep in mind that these charts are for men and women who are 5 feet 8½ inches and in their twenties. Unfortunately, as we age, the distribution of our muscle mass changes, and not to anyone's advantage. After age forty-five, both men and women lose about 10 percent of their lean body mass per decade. That is equivalent to losing about one-third of a pound to half a pound of muscle each year and gaining that much in body fat. The bottom line: whether you're a man or a woman, the older you get, the fewer calories you burn. The good news is that exercise, especially resistance training, can preserve and even increase lean body mass.

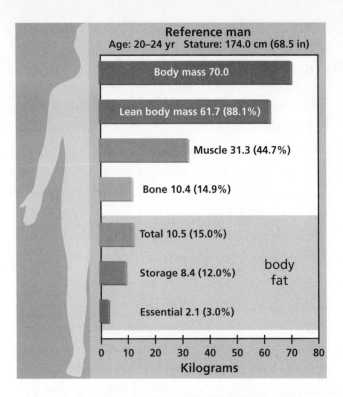

Reference man
Age: 20–24 yr   Stature: 174.0 cm (68.5 in)

Body mass 70.0
Lean body mass 61.7 (88.1%)
Muscle 31.3 (44.7%)
Bone 10.4 (14.9%)
Total 10.5 (15.0%)
Storage 8.4 (12.0%)
body fat
Essential 2.1 (3.0%)

0 10 20 30 40 50 60 70 80
Kilograms

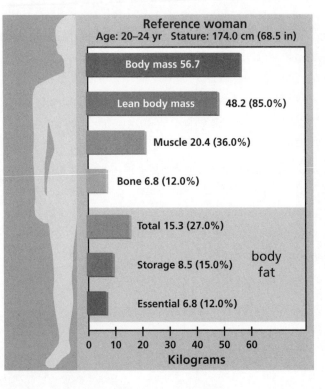

Reference woman
Age: 20–24 yr   Stature: 174.0 cm (68.5 in)

Body mass 56.7
Lean body mass 48.2 (85.0%)
Muscle 20.4 (36.0%)
Bone 6.8 (12.0%)
Total 15.3 (27.0%)
Storage 8.5 (15.0%)
body fat
Essential 6.8 (12.0%)

0 10 20 30 40 50 60
Kilograms

Behnke's theoretical model for the reference man and reference woman. Values in parenthesis represent the specific value expressed as a percentage of total body mass.

Wrapping Things Up

Men and women think about weight gain and loss from different vantage points because each gender experiences them differently physically and emotionally.

- *When* weight gain occurs is typically at different times during adulthood. Women usually gain weight earlier and are especially vulnerable during both the childbirth and childrearing years and menopause. With men, weight gain is more likely to creep up, and most guys often don't notice the extra pounds until there are a lot of them.

- *Why* men and women think weight gain occurs is generally different. Unlike women, men don't equate overeating with negative emotional states. Rather, it's the feel-good emotions and circumstances that are more related to overeating: Men love food and love to eat, especially when they are enjoying themselves. However, when men are asked to explain why they think they've gained weight, they are less likely to see eating too much as the sole (or even the main) cause, and they are more likely to say that it's a matter of genetics or lack of exercise. Women, on the other hand, are much more likely to believe that their excess weight is in large part the result of eating in response to negative emotions. Food provides comfort when things are not going well.

- *How* men and women gain and lose weight is also very different. Men are born with a physical calorie-burning advantage—they have more lean body mass than women, and that enables them to burn more calories even when they're sleeping. But men may also burn more calories because they tend to be more active than women.

Let's Talk!

Looking for ways to understand the past as a means of building a healthy-weight future? Go on a walk and explore the following topics:

1. When did you first notice that you had gained weight?

2. Why do you think you gained weight?

3. What do you think is the best way to lose weight? Why?

CHAPTER 6

Dress Sizes, Belt Notches, and Other Weight-Loss Triggers

Why We Lose Weight

Liberty Central High School's twenty-year class reunion is just weeks away. High school sweethearts Maria and Juan were thrilled when the invitation to their class reunion arrived. In the old days, Maria was a cheerleader, and Juan played the bass drum in the marching band. They both had many friends back in Miami, but Juan's job required that they relocate to Texas. Now they keep in touch with everyone mainly by phone and e-mail. In fact, they figured it had been at least 10 years since they had seen most of their high school pals. Maria and Juan agreed it was time to go back and visit.

While Maria was looking forward to seeing her old friends, she was also nervous. Since getting married and having three children, she had likened her weight to an elevator, always going up and down. The night after making flight and hotel reservations, Maria stepped on the bathroom scale and quickly did the math: She was at least 25 pounds heavier than she had been in high school. Maria had always been athletic and conscientious about what she ate. But between her part-time job, volunteer work, and the kids' school and sports schedules, her eating habits had slipped. Discouraged by her weight, she searched the Internet for the latest ideas on how to lose weight before the reunion. Armed with a new sense of purpose and motivation, she said, "I can't go back and let my friends see me like this! I am going to lose this weight. Starting tomorrow, no more desserts. I'm cutting back on how much I eat and I'm going to walk every day."

Like Maria, Juan was looking forward to going back and reconnecting with his old buddies. Although he, too, had picked up several pounds since high school, he wasn't especially concerned about what people would think about his appearance. He was very concerned about his weight, though. The week before, he had applied for a new life insurance policy and it required him to have a comprehensive physical examination. Much to his surprise, he found out that he had high blood pressure and borderline-high blood sugar. Concerned about his health, Juan had called his doctor and seen him the next day. The doctor told Juan that he needed to take medication to lower his blood pressure, but that if he lost weight, he might be able to reduce or go off the medication and there was a good chance his blood sugar would return to within the normal range. Given the bad news about his health and higher insurance rates, Juan also found himself suddenly motivated to lose weight. That night at dinner he turned to Maria for help: He said, "I know you want to lose weight before we go to the reunion. I need to lose some weight, too. Can you help me? The doctor told me that I need to lose at least twenty pounds if I hope to get off the blood pressure medication. I love you and the kids and I want to be around for a long time. I am going to lose this weight for good!"

Here we have two people, a husband and wife. Both know that they are overweight and both suddenly want to do something about it. Although their goals may be the same—to lose weight—that is where their similarities end. Their motivation for losing weight happens to be very different. Whether it is a high school reunion or hypertension, before most people voluntarily commit themselves to losing weight, something triggers the motivation. Like Maria, many women are initially motivated to take off extra pounds because they want to look better. While appearance is important to guys, too, it's often the diagnosis of a health problem like Juan's that makes them get serious about losing weight.

Not only do different reasons often motivate women and men to start losing weight, but what motivates anyone to continue losing weight after the first days also tends to change and shift. Studies have discovered that motivations generally change from the beginning to the end of weight loss and beyond. A continuing desire to achieve a healthy weight is key to lasting weight loss. This chapter sheds some light on what makes women and men want to start losing and what then keeps them motivated to achieve lasting results.

Sparking People's Interest in Losing Weight

Before making a serious commitment to weight loss, most people have some sort of experience or trigger that gets them fired up and ready to begin. Whereas the details of the experience vary, two motivators of weight loss remain fundamental: appearance and health. Both are important to men and women alike, although there tends to be some gender and age differences when it comes to just how much each factor contributes to the weight-loss equation.

Let's start with appearance. Studies have found that the primary trigger setting off most women's decision to lose weight has to do with appearance. Thin is in, and losing weight makes most women feel more attractive. And that is fine as long as a woman has excess weight to lose or has been putting on pounds that she didn't have as a twenty-year-old. If, however, excess weight is not an issue, then weight loss may be an attempt to alleviate issues of poor self-esteem or a distorted body image. Losing weight in this situation is not a good idea.

When does a woman know that the time is right for an appearance-related weight-loss effort? It generally boils down to one of two triggers. The first is when clothing no longer fits. When a woman goes up a dress size or can no longer breathe comfortably in her jeans, she's often motivated to start losing weight. Social situations are the second trigger that women cite as a motivator to get started losing weight. Special events, like a class reunion or a wedding, are likely to jump-start a woman's enthusiasm to lose weight, often playing a greater role in women's motivation than in men's.

As we discussed in chapter 3, women, when they are in the public eye, are more likely than men to be concerned with how others view them, especially in relation to their physical appearance and their weight. Special events are a prime example of being in the public eye. Knowing that a special event may be an emotionally vulnerable time, many women prepare for the event by deciding to lose weight to improve their appearance.

Men care about their appearance, too. But for men more than for women, age seems to be a greater factor in the way appearance works to trigger weight loss. Weight Watchers research has found that men under the age of forty-five are far more likely than older men to say that their primary reason for losing weight is to look better or to get more fit. And when those guys are asked to give more details about their experience, another difference between the genders emerges. Men nearly always cite a situation involving clothing as the deciding point for taking action. Pants that are too tight and the need to go up a belt notch are the most often heard triggers. Unlike women, many men are simply not motivated to lose weight by special events that will put them in the public spotlight. Men believe that they are more likely to be judged on factors other than weight during such social occasions.

Weight loss isn't just about appearance. Health is a real motivator as well, especially for older men. Several clinical studies have found that health seems to be the primary trigger setting off most men's decision to lose weight. Weight Watchers research confirms that existing health problems seem to top many men's list of reasons for wanting to lose weight. Some of the most common health problems men said that they hope to reduce or eliminate with weight loss include type 2 diabetes, high blood pressure, elevated blood lipids, sleep apnea, digestive problems, back problems, and joint pain. How do most guys become aware of the fact that they have health problems? Usually their doctors tell them. One Weight Watchers Online subscriber summed it up rather frankly when he stated, "The doctor said my diabetes and high blood pressure can be controlled for maybe one more year without my losing weight. It's lose weight or die."

Men aren't the only ones motivated to lose weight for health reasons—women are, too—but the key difference between the genders is in the timing. Whereas men are more likely to be motivated because they want to fix existing health problems, women are more likely to lose weight to prevent the health problems from occurring in the first place.

Is there a preferred trigger to cause a person to make the decision to lose weight? No. Whether the inspiration comes from a desire to improve one's appearance or enhance one's health, what's crucial is that the inspiration is important enough to motivate action. The take-home message when losing weight as a couple is to remember that weight-loss triggers are very personal. What inspires one person can make no impression on the other, so trying to persuade someone to lose weight for a reason that's important to you is unlikely to be effective.

FROM A WOMAN'S VIEWPOINT
SPARKING PEOPLE'S INTEREST IN LOSING WEIGHT

Women tend to be more emotionally tuned into their weight, which can be a good thing if they are overweight as it helps them to become more aware and to take action to lose weight. But some women may become too emotional about their weight, and that mind-set can affect their mental well-being. Research has found that there is a relationship between depression and obesity and that obese women are much more likely than obese men to be severely depressed. Conversely, lasting weight loss is linked to lower levels of depression. When depression and excess weight are coexisting issues, many experts recommend that they seek treatment for each.

FROM A MAN'S VIEWPOINT
SPARKING PEOPLE'S INTEREST IN LOSING WEIGHT

Weight Watchers research has found that men are much less likely than women to dwell on their weight. They are also less likely to say that they are completely dissatisfied with their weight or extremely bothered by it. Although not allowing excess weight to become an emotional burden is good, having no emotional connection to it can have drawbacks, especially for those with a lot of weight to lose. It is human nature for people to take a committed action in response to those things they care about deeply. Caring is an emotion, and a lack of caring or not caring enough about weight may prevent some men from doing what it takes to lose the extra pounds.

REAL-LIFE LESSONS
Wedding Bells and Weight-Loss Blues

Situation: Our only daughter is getting married later this year and my husband and I are planning the wedding. I knew that I was overweight, but I wanted to look good in the pictures. So I started to eat less, and I've been able to lose about twenty pounds. My husband needs to lose weight, too. He says that he's trying, but I don't see any progress. Why won't he try harder?

Strategies: The decision to take the plunge and commit oneself to losing weight is a very personal one. Clearly, your daughter's wedding is an effective trigger for you. Just as clearly, the event does not send "Lose Weight Now!" signals to your husband, and there is nothing you can do to change that. If your husband is simply not interested in losing weight now, your best bet is to leave him alone. Bugging him will only annoy him and may even make him more resistant to doing something. If, however, he's expressing an interest in losing weight but the upcoming wedding isn't the motivator to make it happen, try to find a trigger that will help him make the leap. Perhaps offering to take full charge of the food preparation or asking him to join you in a physical activity will make a difference. If not, simply stay with your commitment and enjoy the success. It is possible that when your husband sees you dancing at your daughter's wedding with wonderful energy while he has to take frequent breaks from the action, that will be just what he needs to decide to shed the weight.

What You Know Matters

How many calories are in a slice of pizza? Which is more filling, brown rice or white rice? When trying to lose weight, knowledge is power. Knowing about nutrition and how eating affects health allows a person a great deal of freedom and flexibility when making choices about food. It appears that knowledge can also influence people's motivation to lose weight.

Based on both scientific and market research, we can conclude that women currently have the nutrition-information advantage over guys, regardless of their weight status. For example, when researchers in England assessed the nutrition knowledge of over 1,000 men and women to help determine people's understanding of the current dietary recommendations, the most healthful food choices, and diet–disease links, they discovered that in general the women in the study had more such knowledge than the men.

Why do women appear to be more nutrition-savvy than men? Part of the answer may lie in the mass media—television, radio, newspapers, and magazines. For the past several decades, women have been the primary target of publicized information on health and nutrition. That means that health news stories and health campaigns have been developed to be more appealing and more intriguing to women than to men.

Being exposed so often to messages about obesity, health, and nutrition may have helped women keep the need for a healthy lifestyle in mind and may have influenced their decision to lose weight. Although knowledge in itself doesn't guarantee behavior change, it does appear to make a difference. In a Swedish study that examined the lifestyle differences in over 4,000 men and women, the women showed more interest in measures of health prevention. They also tended to have a healthier lifestyle than the men. The women in the study were less likely to be overweight or obese, and compared with the men, they consumed significantly more vegetables, fruits, and milk and less meat, fat, and alcohol.

If knowledge is power and more is better when it comes to weight loss, can knowledge about nutrition affect the food choices that men make? One study, done in France, seems to point in that direction. It involved more than 350 men between the ages of forty-five and sixty-four. The men were given a quiz that assessed nutrition knowledge. The researchers found that those men with the highest scores made healthier food choices than those with the lowest scores. In particular, the high-scoring men consumed less fat and less animal fat. Since a high-fat diet is associated with excess weight and consequent health problems, the findings from this study are encouraging.

FROM A WOMAN'S VIEWPOINT
WHAT YOU KNOW MATTERS

The media have certainly helped provide women with a plethora of health and nutrition information. Women today are better educated about health issues than women of any previous generation. But things can get confusing when reliable health and wellness information gets mixed up with unconstructive images that support an unhealthy lifestyle. Just as women are media targets for good information, they are also repeatedly exposed to images of underweight models and messages that erode self-esteem. That negative information has the potential to increase negative moods, dissatisfaction with one's body, and possibly the symptoms of an eating disorder. Some studies have correlated a greater exposure to the mass media (television, movies, magazines, and the Internet) with a higher probability of obesity and a negative body image.

FROM A MAN'S VIEWPOINT
WHAT YOU KNOW MATTERS

Compared with what's available to women, far fewer media resources specifically target men with accurate nutrition and health information. So whom or what do guys turn to for help in finding nutrition and weight-loss information? According to Weight Watchers research, men go to the people they perceive as experts. First and most importantly men seek out the women in their lives as their preferred experts for weight-loss help. Men also seek expert advice from their doctors. Given the paucity of nutrition information specifically targeted at men, it appears that the media have an opportunity to reach them with key nutrition and health information about their need to lose weight and the benefits to be gained by doing so.

REAL-LIFE LESSONS
Finding Accurate Weight-Loss Information

Situation: Whenever I have a question about weight loss, I ask my wife because I trust her. She says she doesn't mind my asking, but I feel as if I need some other in-depth resources. Any suggestions?

Strategies: Getting reliable advice and information about weight loss is critical to lasting success, yet sometimes it can be tough because there is so much information out there that ranges from excellent to mediocre to downright hazardous to your health! Seeking out a source that you trust makes sense. On the Internet there are several sites sponsored by government agencies and professional organizations that provide excellent general information that you may find useful. For specific guidance and expertise, you might want to look to Weight Watchers. Attending a Weight Watchers meeting will give you direct access to a weight-loss expert. All Weight Watchers leaders have achieved a healthy body weight by following the Weight Watchers program and are keeping the weight off the same way. They have received extensive training about the program and are motivated to help you achieve the same success they are enjoying. While you may think that Weight Watchers meetings are just for women, think again. Men are regular attendees—hundreds of thousands go to Weight Watchers meetings each year—and like the women who attend, they value the information and expertise they receive in the weekly meetings. In addition to Weight Watchers meetings, WeightWatchers.com provides a vast amount of expert information. Weight Watchers also offers Weight Watchers Online, a subscription product designed for self-helpers, with Internet tools and resources to assist with weight-loss efforts. As you seek out and find the expertise that helps you, be sure to share your newfound knowledge with your wife. I'm sure she'll appreciate it.

Audrey and Norm Parker
PENNSYLVANIA

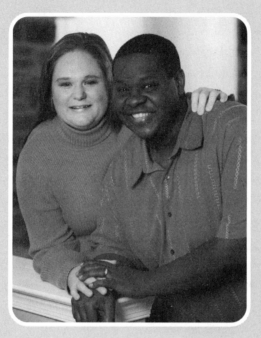

Audrey, who is in her late twenties, and Norm, who is in his mid-thirties, have been married for a little over a year. They met each other about five years ago while working at the same chemical company. Audrey is a plant engineer and Norm works in purchasing.

Audrey was a Division I college athlete. She was on the track team and threw the discus and the shot put. Audrey explained, "I never had problems with my weight before because I was always working out." But after college she met Norm, and while they were dating they both slowly but steadily gained weight. After becoming engaged, the pending nuptials acted as a wake-up call. Audrey found herself 50 pounds heavier than she had been in college. She explains, "I did not feel comfortable with myself anymore. I went through my wardrobe and nothing fit. What really scared me was that I could no longer shop in regular stores. I had to go to places that carried extra and plus sizes."

On New Year's Eve, Audrey and Norm agreed to lose weight before the wedding. While Audrey was determined, Norm was skeptical. According to Norm, "I have always been heavy, and any time I tried to lose weight, it never seemed to work." At the end of January, a friend asked Audrey to join her in signing up for Weight Watchers at Work, and since she didn't have a plan for losing the weight, she decided to give it a try. "At first, Norm wouldn't sign up with me because he didn't think it would work for someone like him, meaning a guy," said Audrey. But despite Norm's skepticism, both of them began to benefit from Audrey's decision. They were eating the same healthy foods and going on daily walks together. By July, Norm found himself 44 pounds lighter and a firm believer that Weight Watchers works for guys, so he joined Audrey's At Work Group. They both followed the Flex Plan and found it helpful and easy to use. By their wedding day in November, Norm and Audrey were a combined 90 pounds lighter.

After their wedding, Audrey's motivation to continue losing weight was her hope of someday having a child. She explains, "I had heard from so many women at our Weight Watchers meetings that they gained most of their weight after having children. I wanted to get my weight down so that I would be able to avoid that problem." And it's good that she did, as Audrey has just found out that she is pregnant with their first child. She says, "I know I can't lose weight right now, but Weight Watchers has taught me how to eat healthier. I plan to go back to Weight Watchers as soon as the baby is born and I can rejoin my group."

Meanwhile, Norm is continuing to lose weight. "The weight has come off so fast!" he says. "It seems as if every month or so I am tightening my belt a notch, and my shirt size keeps going down. I never knew there were stores for guys other than the big and tall kinds." In addition to looking better, Norm has discovered that his health problems are also disappearing. He no longer has to wear a sleep apnea mask at night, and his blood pressure medication has been reduced. According to Norm, "My new motivation is my child. I want to be able to chase him or her around and not be out of breath."

Audrey and Norm feel that joining Weight Watchers and losing weight together have been the keys to their success. When Audrey said that she might have been able to lose the weight on her own, Norm said, "No way!" They agreed that losing weight with each other has made it much more fun and definitely easier.

How to Stay Motivated and Keep on Losing

What motivates people to start losing weight is often not enough to *keep* them motivated. As weight loss progresses, new reasons to continue are often needed. Both women and men seem to be spurred on by seeing the physical results of weight loss, but many women also need more in terms of positive emotional feedback in order to reach their ultimate weight goals.

Based on Weight Watchers research, we conclude that men whose weight loss is triggered by a health problem tend to become even more motivated when they see the positive physical effects that come with weight loss. Lowering blood pressure, dropping a couple of pounds a week, no longer needing to take medicine for diabetes—all those results seem to rev guys up and make them want to keep losing. And what's particularly inspirational for guys (but not so much for women) is the immediate gratification they often get from physical results. That's because, as we learned in chapter 5, men are biologically programmed to lose more weight than women and to lose it at a faster rate. And since many of the health problems men experience are improved by losing weight (sometimes as little as 10 pounds), they often get quicker results and therefore more positive reinforcement.

Like men, women are also motivated by successful physical results such as lowered blood pressure or blood sugar, particularly if preventing or alleviating a health problem triggered their commitment to losing weight in the first place. But seeing the needle on the scale go down is what seems to keep most women motivated. Because it often takes women a bit longer to lose weight than men, though, many women need something else to keep their weight-loss motivation high—women need to feel better emotionally, too. Since women tend to be emotionally tuned into their weight and are concerned about how others view them, they are often motivated by positive feedback. Women thrive on recognition or acknowledgment from

others—a spouse, friends, coworkers, and others—tha⟩
ing weight and that they are doing well. Most women re
ing compliments about how much thinner they look. ⟩
certainly enjoy receiving compliments and public rec
feedback doesn't appear to be as great a motivator for them as it is for
women.

Willpower: Weight-Loss Fact or Myth?

How many times have you ever heard this before: "If she'd simply stop herself from eating so much, she wouldn't have a
weight problem"? Or how about this one: "If he'd just make
himself go to the gym every day, he'd get rid of that belly"?
Many people mistakenly believe that a lack of willpower is the
sole reason everyone is overweight. In fact, a Weight Watchers
survey of its members found that 50 percent of women and
men believe that willpower is all you need to lose weight. The
truth is that willpower is only part of what it takes. Losing
weight and keeping it off require more than willpower; they
require a comprehensive weight-loss plan that includes maintaining a positive mind-set, paying attention to food choices,
getting regular physical activity, and creating a supportive
atmosphere.

FROM A WOMAN'S VIEWPOINT
HOW TO STAY MOTIVATED AND KEEP ON LOSING

Weight Watchers conducted a study to learn more about women's and
men's attitudes about what it takes to lose weight. They discovered
that one of the main differences between women and men has to do
with dieting: women said they were "sick of doing it," but men did not
have a similar reaction. Chances are that the typical woman has made
a lot more weight-loss attempts than the average guy. But women

should hang in there because they are headed down the right weight-loss path. The reality is that the only way to lose weight is to eat less and, as the extra pounds disappear, continue to watch what you eat and exercise.

FROM A MAN'S VIEWPOINT
HOW TO STAY MOTIVATED AND KEEP ON LOSING

According to a Weight Watchers study, while women said they were tired of dieting, men did not. Given that men prefer to exercise rather than restrict their eating, that is not that surprising. Studies also show that fewer men than women diet. The problem with the exercise-only approach, though, is that if guys want to lose more weight, they are going to need to bite the bullet and start taking in fewer calories—that's the only way to lose a substantial amount of weight.

REAL-LIFE LESSONS
Staying Motivated

Situation: My entire family is going on a cruise next week: husband, kids, grandparents, siblings—everyone! Last year when I found out we were going, I started trying to lose weight. So far I've lost about 50 pounds, but I have 15 more to go. I know I will probably gain a few pounds on the cruise, but I'm not sure how to get back on track after we return. Any thoughts?

Strategies: You are smart to realize that the cruise is likely to put your weight loss on hold for a week. Rather than abandon all efforts, however, why not strive to return from the cruise at the same weight you left home? Walking the deck, taking physically active side trips, and making wise food choices at mealtime may be effective ways to take a break from your weight-loss regimen without experiencing a backslide. If you can achieve that goal, you're likely to return from your week away with a sense of pride and accomplishment, which in turn can fuel your commitment to losing more weight. Sometimes taking a break—without abandoning your efforts—can be a good thing as it allows you a bit of a breather to recharge your batteries, bask in the success that you've already had, and regroup for the future.

Wrapping Things Up

Something needs to spark or trigger a person's decision to start losing weight. As weight loss progresses, new motivators are often needed.

- Women and younger men are often initially motivated to lose weight by a concern about their appearance. Clothes becoming too small is an effective trigger in both sexes, whereas special events, like a class reunion or an anniversary party, are often all it takes to spring a woman into weight-loss mode. Older guys, on the other hand, are more likely to be motivated to lose weight for health reasons. A doctor's diagnosis of a health problem is a frequent catalyst for men to take weight-loss action.

- Knowledge is power when it comes to weight loss. Knowing what to do helps people feel more in control and more confident. Currently women are generally more knowledgeable than men about health, nutrition, and how eating affects weight loss; consequently, according to studies on the subject, women in general seem to have healthier eating habits than men. However, given that men have historically been the target of less media-disseminated nutrition information, it stands to reason that they will benefit from knowing more about healthy eating and strategies for losing weight when going forward.

- Getting started is only one aspect of losing weight. Everyone needs to stay motivated until all of the weight is lost. What sustains weight-loss motivation is a bit different for women and men. Men are usually bolstered by positive physical results, such as lower blood sugar readings, lower cholesterol levels, or reductions in medication for a weight-related health problem. On the other hand, the motivation for women is usually a little more complex. That's because it's often tied to both physical results—losing pounds—and emotional feedback, recognition, and compliments from others. Women often need both to spur them on to losing weight.

Let's Talk!

Before attempting to lose weight, think through the following questions so that you can start out strong and stay fired up until you have achieved all of your weight-loss goals:

1. What would it take for you to become seriously motivated to start losing weight?

2. Do you feel you have enough nutrition information to make the food choices that will best help you lose weight successfully?

3. While losing weight, how do you plan on staying motivated?

CHAPTER 7

How We Lose Weight

The Two Sexes Do It Differently

Surprise! Jeff quickly surveys his apartment and is shocked to see it jam-packed with neighbors, close friends, and family members. His younger sister, Traci, thought it would be a great idea to throw a party for Jeff's fortieth birthday. About a year ago, Jeff went through a painful divorce, and he has had a hard time getting his life back in order. He's become a workaholic—he rarely goes out and makes no attempt to date. Traci suspects that his behavior might have something to do with the fact that he has put on a lot of weight, especially around his stomach.

Toward the end of the party, several of Jeff's friends urge him to open his gifts. Reluctantly Jeff unwraps the usual age-related gag gifts—fiber supplements and adult diapers. A gift from his cousin Jill attracts his attention: the latest diet book, *How to Lose 20 Pounds in 2 Weeks and Feel Like You're 20*. Traci, who has been trying to lose weight on and off since she was a teenager, thinks it is the perfect gift. She says, "Jill! Where on earth did you find that book? I've been looking for it forever. It's been on back-order for months. All the talk show hosts and magazines have given it rave reviews. All you have to do is follow the hourly meal plans and do all your grocery shopping online. Then you can use your cell phone to log in with a personal eating plan consultant. I can't wait to read that book!"

Jeff, who has been listening intently to his sister, takes a few minutes to flip through the book. He grasps that it's over 300 pages and full of lists of all sorts. He says, "Jill, this looks complicated, but it looks like something I can use. Traci, why don't you read it first? Then you can fill me in on what I need to do!"

How to lose weight? It's a topic that women and men share an interest in. But knowing that weight loss is needed is one thing, and actually losing weight is another. In addition, men and women differ in how often they take action and the general strategies they use. Like Traci, women are more likely than men to start a weight-loss plan. Many women have a long history of trying a variety of diets and weight-loss approaches. Perhaps because of their varied experience, they tend to want to know all the details before they make the decision to try a new approach—what, how much, and when they will eat; how much weight they can expect to lose; how much it will cost; and whether they need to exercise. Armed with that knowledge, the typical woman will then discuss the approach with others to get their opinions and thoughts on the topic before getting started.

Most men, on the other hand, respond more the way Jeff did. Part of the reason is that the average guy, generally speaking, has less experience with a variety of weight-loss approaches than his female friends. When most guys are deciding to lose weight, they are less likely to amass a lot of detailed information or compare the specifics of various dieting methods. They are also less likely to ask a bunch of people for their opinion of which method to use. Instead, men tend to focus on the basics of the approach—what they can and cannot do. With that information in hand and perhaps after a consultation with someone he considers a weight-loss expert, the typical man will start. Then, as he is losing weight and seeing progress, he will get more information, and as he gains experience with the method, he will explore it in more detail.

Trying to get a man to lose weight the way a woman does is unlikely to succeed. Likewise, women do not respond well to a man's way of losing weight. This chapter will help women and men appreciate that there is no right approach to deciding what weight-loss method to follow. The important thing to remember is that both women and men can achieve successful weight loss if they take the time to consider their different perspectives and support each other's preferred weight-loss approach.

Making the Effort

Given that two-thirds of adult Americans are overweight and five out of the ten leading causes of death in the United States and Canada (heart disease, cancer, stroke, diabetes, and kidney disease) are associated with being overweight, weight loss is an issue that both women and men must face.

Many adults have a fair amount of experience when trying to lose weight. Here are some of the findings from four U.S. surveys that have looked at the health practices of men and women:

- 33 to 40 percent of adult women are working to lose weight, and 20 to 24 percent of adult men are doing so.

- 28 percent of both men and women said that they were working to maintain their current weight.

- Over the past year, women who work at trying to lose weight report spending an average of 6.4 months in the effort; men say that they spent an average of 5.8 months.

- Over a two-year period, the average woman says that she's made 2.5 weight-loss attempts; the average man indicates that he made 2.

- Among those working to lose weight, 84 percent of women and 76 percent of men reported following a low-calorie diet, and 60 percent of both men and women reported increasing their physical activity.

What do these numbers mean? First, the percentage of people actively engaged in weight loss is quite low compared with the numbers who are overweight and obese. This is particularly true for men. Second, the statistics indicate that most people's attempts at weight loss are an on-again, off-again experience as opposed to an ongoing effort using a lifestyle approach. Finally, many people have a tendency to make a choice either to restrict food or to exercise as the means to achieve success, but not both.

Clearly, achieving lasting weight loss needs to be a priority to stem the growing rates of overweight and obesity among men and women. It's apparent that there is much room for improvement in the approaches that both women and men take to make that happen.

FROM A WOMAN'S VIEWPOINT
MAKING THE EFFORT

Women tend to accumulate more weight loss experience than men. As the surveys discussed above show, women are more likely to be working at weight loss at any given time, they make more attempts per year, and they spend more time in each attempt. But there is another fact that adds to women's experience with weight loss: they tend to start younger. According to a U.S. National Institutes of Health report, when a nationally representative sample of high school students was given a self-administered questionnaire, 44 percent of the female students and 15 percent of the male students reported that they were trying to lose weight; another 26 percent of the female students said that they were working to keep from gaining weight as compared with 15 percent of the male students.

The impact of all that weight-loss experience is difficult to evaluate and depends a lot on the individual. As the saying goes, there is no better teacher than experience, and trying different weight-loss approaches can provide valuable lessons in what works and what doesn't. On the other hand, repeated attempts at losing weight with ineffective approaches can lead to frustration, discouragement, and the decision to stop trying. Picking a comprehensive weight-management approach with proven results makes the most sense for a woman wanting to lose weight, regardless of her level of experience.

FROM A MAN'S VIEWPOINT
MAKING THE EFFORT

The survey just mentioned didn't look at the genders by age, and Weight Watchers research indicates that age may be an important factor. Research done for Weight Watchers has found that men under the age of forty-five are gaining weight at a younger age than their fathers and grandfathers. They are more concerned about their appearance and their health, and they are thinking about taking action to lose weight. Younger men were more likely than men over the age of forty-five to state that they expected to follow a structured eating plan in the next 6 months.

REAL-LIFE LESSON
All Talk and No Weight-Loss Action

Situation: My wife and I have been married for seven years. Her weight is driving me crazy! It seems as if she's always talking about losing weight, but from what I can tell, she isn't doing anything—she keeps getting heavier. When I tell her what I think she should do, she becomes angry and accuses me of being insensitive and uncaring. I do care! My wife has gained 75 pounds since we have been married, and I would like the woman I married to return. How can I help her lose weight?

Strategies: It looks as if you're experiencing one of the major differences in how men and women approach weight loss. Women like your wife tend to work through their decision to lose weight in a verbal way. In other words, she's thinking out loud. In order to make the leap to lasting weight loss, she needs to go through the stages of thinking and then planning before she will be truly ready to take action. Men, on the other hand, tend to do their thinking and planning silently, verbalizing their decision to lose weight only as they are acting on it. Telling your wife to take action now is not working because she's not yet at the stage where she's ready to do that. To help her get there, accept that she needs to think and plan. When she talks about losing weight, ask her a few questions that might help her find her way. For example, is a lack of confidence a problem? If so, reinforce the idea that she can successfully lose weight and remind her that you'll be there to help her every step of the way. Does she have other priorities that are keeping her desire to lose weight at the bottom of her to-do list? Helping her sort through those other priorities—whether they involve the desire to be the perfect parent, keep an immaculate home, or advance in a job—may help her move weight loss closer to the top of her list.

You'll know that your wife has moved from thinking to planning when she starts to talk about specific weight-loss methods. Rather than give her your opinion of what will work, ask her about the pros and cons, and challenge her to find ways to overcome the probable barriers before getting started. Listening to your wife and assessing where she is in her approach to weight loss will provide you with insights that will allow you to help her get to the place where she needs to be to make weight loss a reality.

How Women and Men Decide What They'll Do

The thought processes and the logic used to arrive at a decision about what weight-loss approach to take tends to be different for women and men. Most women prefer diplomacy; they want to have in-depth discussions with a variety of people and explore as many solutions as possible. Most men, on the other hand, declare war. Guys are much less inclined to spend a lot of time talking with a lot of people; they prefer to make a decision and act on it.

Before starting a weight-loss program, many women feel compelled to discuss their options and goals with others—men and women. A woman is much more likely than a man to talk for quite some time—weeks, months, even years—about her desire to lose weight. That's because before she makes her final decision, a woman needs to confer with several other people—her spouse or significant other, family members, coworkers, friends, and, most important, other successful "losers" at weight loss. Primarily, they are investigating what weight-loss methods are likely to have the best results for them. For example, it is not uncommon for a woman to ask a coworker who lost a visible amount of weight to share his or her insight on the topic. If the coworker is a woman, most likely she will welcome the opportunity to share her story, and the two women will enter into a long dialogue about what works and what doesn't. If the coworker is a man, he will probably appreciate the fact that the woman noticed his weight loss, but he'll be much less likely to provide a blow-by-blow account of what he's done to achieve it.

Looking at the way many men make their decisions regarding weight can be baffling to women. That's because when a man announces that he is going to get into shape and lose weight, it often takes a woman by surprise; it may even be the first time she has heard him talk about it. What many women don't understand is that most men prefer to solve their problems silently and on their own rather than discuss them with others. So when a man announces his intention to lose weight, it's more than likely that he's been mulling over the decision for some time. In a survey of male users of Weight Watchers Online, the guys reported that the decision to subscribe was not a spur-of-the-moment event but the outcome of a period of dissatisfaction with their weight.

The fact that women and men both eventually make the decision to lose weight and then pick an approach puts them on common ground. What members of the opposite sex need to realize and respect is that the processes each sex uses to arrive at that point are different and serve different purposes.

FROM A WOMAN'S VIEWPOINT
HOW WOMEN AND MEN DECIDE WHAT THEY'LL DO

Most women will be the first to admit that they need the support of others in order to lose weight successfully. Whom or what do women turn to when they need help losing weight? The media, books, and friends.

FROM A MAN'S VIEWPOINT
HOW WOMEN AND MEN DECIDE WHAT THEY'LL DO

The fact that men tend to be more private in making their weight-related decisions doesn't mean that they will not seek out help if they feel that doing so will improve their decision. Rather than talking to a variety of people, however, the typical guy will seek out an expert. According to research conducted for Weight Watchers, men's preferred source for nutrition information is their spouse. It appears that men notice all the research that women do in preparation for losing weight and they respect their wives' opinions and advice—especially if provided in response to their request.

REAL-LIFE LESSON
Too Many Questions!

Situation: My husband is thirty-five years old, holds an MBA, and owns and operates his own business—he is an intelligent, self-motivated man. Unfortunately, he has gained a lot of weight in the fourteen years that we've been married. I lost quite a bit of weight a few years ago and am working hard to keep it off. Last week he told me that he was ready to lose weight and would like to follow the eating plan that I followed to lose my weight. What I can't understand is why he won't take the time to learn about the plan himself. Instead, he keeps firing off questions, like "Can I eat bread?" or "Can I have one chicken thigh or two?" I am getting frustrated with him. It feels as if I'm doing all the work. Any suggestions on how I can get him more involved?

Strategies: While it may be hard to accept, you should see your husband's reliance as a compliment to you and not laziness on his part. Because he sees that you are successfully keeping the weight that you lost off, he believes that you know what you're doing. Hence, he is going to you—the expert—to get the information he needs to get started. As he, too, starts to see success, he will likely want to have a better understanding of the whats and whys of what you're telling him to do. But from his point of view, there's no need to take the time to learn the details until he has a reason (for example, he's having success, wants it to continue, and knows that he'll need to know more than he does now to keep it going). For now, just answer his questions and focus on creating his success. Have faith that in time he will want to know more. When he starts asking more in-depth questions, that will be the time to give him some reading materials.

Shirley Steinke and her son, Allen
COLORADO

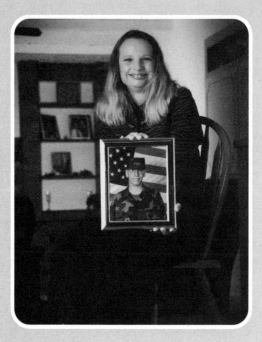

Ever since the 1980s Shirley had been on and off numerous weight-loss plans. "I've tried just about all of them," says Shirley. "They worked for a while, but I'm a picky eater, and I got tired of eating the same foods. Unfortunately, I gained back all the weight I had lost and then added more." Shirley has been married for twenty-seven years to Lee, and they have two grown children, Anna, who is twenty-five years old, and Allen, twenty-two.

Allen, at 6 feet 1, is a big guy. His lifelong dream was to join the military, but at 260 pounds, he was too heavy. The army told him that he needed to get his weight down to at least 210 before he could enlist.

Motivated to lose weight, Allen turned to his mom for help. She explained, "My husband's sister, who lived in Minnesota, lost a lot of weight on Weight Watchers, so I talked with her a lot about the program. I never knew Weight Watchers had more than one eating option to help you lose weight, and I really like the health emphasis, so it seemed like the perfect approach for Allen." Since Shirley wanted to help her son, she decided to give Weight Watchers a try so that they could lose weight together. She says, "Allen preferred the Core Plan, which allowed him to focus on a list of wholesome, nutritious foods and didn't require him to count anything. I, on the other hand, loved the Flex Plan because I was free to eat what I wanted as long as I counted my **POINTS**® values."

With Weight Watchers, Allen and Shirley started steadily losing weight: Allen lost about 2 pounds a week; Shirley lost about 1 pound a week. It took a little over 1 year for Allen to lose his weight, 60 pounds. He was able to enlist in the army and went to Iraq in 2005. Now stationed in Oklahoma, he is a specialist driving trucks. Shirley also lost about twenty-eight pounds and was so excited about her success that she began working as a receptionist for Weight Watchers in Colorado.

Shirley and Allen's weight-loss success was contagious. After observing their tremendous results and seeing how tasty the meals they prepared were, both Lee and Anna decided to give Weight Watchers a try. They both lost weight and are now Lifetime members. According to Shirley, "We all needed to lose weight and eat healthier. Weight Watchers has taught my whole family to eat better." Shirley's blood cholesterol, which was always on the high side, is now under 200, and everyone in the family is slimmer, including Shirley's mother-in-law, who started last year.

Women's and Men's Preferred Weight-Loss Approaches

A key decision that both men and women face after making a commitment to lose weight is the approach—a structured eating plan, an exercise regimen, or a combination of the two—that they are going to follow. Many women have a tendency to be bottom-up thinkers, which means that they want to understand all the details about a weight-loss plan before getting started—that way they can put all the pieces together and see the bigger picture. Men, however, are more likely to be top-down thinkers and prefer to view the big picture first and be briefed on the details later. In other words, when selecting a weight-loss program, women are more likely to want to know the whole story and read the full report, whereas men want to begin with the summary.

Why do most women opt to know all the details before undertaking a weight-loss effort? Part of the answer may lie in the fact that the typical woman has a fair amount of weight-loss experience. Because she's already tried a variety of approaches, a woman may have a greater desire to know the nitty-gritty nuances of a weight-loss method. Armed with that knowledge, she will feel better informed and more confident about making the right choice. Among the details women are interested in are how many calories the weight-loss plan allows, how much and how quickly weight will be lost, whether specific foods must be eaten or avoided, and whether the eating plan or the exercise plan will have any adverse effects on the body (diarrhea, constipation, low blood sugar, sore muscles, and so on). If a weight-loss plan meets with a woman's approval, she will proceed with caution. Only after a woman has experienced some success will she be willing to let go some of the details; at that point she trusts that what she is doing is working.

The level of detail that most women seek before starting a weight-loss plan can be a turnoff for many men. That's because once guys have made the decision to lose weight, they want to get started and all they need are the basics; theirs is a "just tell me what to do" approach.

In a Weight Watchers study looking at approaches to weight loss, 79 percent of the men surveyed said that they simply wanted practical weight-loss information ("just give me the facts"). However, as men begin to follow a weight-loss plan and are successful at losing weight, their interest in knowing more of the details is piqued.

The following breakfast conversation illustrates how a woman and a man on a structured eating plan might communicate using their details versus facts perspectives.

He says: "Breakfast—I'm starved! Yes or no: Can I have eggs?"

She says: "Yes, you can have eggs. In fact, you can have them poached, hard-boiled, scrambled with fat-free milk, or fried with no more than one-half teaspoon of oil."

He says: "I think I'll make a poached egg. Would you like one? And by the way, can I have a piece of toast?"

She says: "No, thanks, on the egg. I think I'll have a six-ounce carton of fat-free yogurt instead, so that I can get a start on my daily calcium recommendation. And yes, you can have toast, but it has to be whole wheat, and you can put one teaspoon of sugar-free jam on top."

He says: "I am so glad you know all of this. It's a lot of information to keep straight.

She says: "Don't worry. You'll get used to it."

You probably noticed that the woman seemed to be totally into the plan, while the man seemed more hesitant because of all the details. Despite the fact that both men and women want to lose weight, they may need to use different approaches in order to meet with weight-loss success. A woman may want to choose an approach that provides details about what, when, and how things should be done. Many men may be better off with an approach that focuses on fewer details while still getting the job done.

FROM A WOMAN'S VIEWPOINT
WOMEN'S AND MEN'S PREFERRED WEIGHT-LOSS APPROACHES

One of the reasons that many women seem to be more actively involved with losing weight is that they are willing to keep trying different approaches until they find a solution that works for them. Weight Watchers studies over the years have found that to be true. Female members consistently report trying several more weight-loss approaches before joining Weight Watchers than male members do.

FROM A MAN'S VIEWPOINT
WOMEN'S AND MEN'S PREFERRED WEIGHT-LOSS APPROACHES

Compared with women, many men tend to have more of a delayed reaction when attempting weight loss. But once guys make the decision to lose weight, they commit themselves and are more likely than women to adhere strictly to a weight-loss plan. For example, 64 percent of male subscribers to Weight Watchers Online reported full compliance with the food plan, a significantly higher percentage than that reported by their female counterparts.

REAL-LIFE LESSON
Finding the Right Approach

Situation: My wife and I are both trying to lose weight. She spent a lot of time trying to find the best weight-loss program so that we could do this together. We have been following the meal plans and both of us have lost some weight. But I am getting really tired of having to make so many food choices and paying such close attention to how much I eat. However, my wife loves it, and it seems to be perfect for her. Is there an approach that might work better for me?

Strategies: The saying "different strokes for different folks" is certainly true when it comes to eating for weight loss. That's why Weight Watchers offers two approaches. So ask your wife and yourself this question: When it comes to my diet, how do I define freedom? Is it being free to eat any food that I want yet knowing that I will need to keep track of my choices so that I'll still be losing weight? Or is freedom eating from a list of wholesome, nutritious foods so that I am satisfied and losing weight without the need to keep track? Sounds as though your wife would say yes to the first part of the question and you would say yes to the second part. The good news is that you can both get what you want. The Flex Plan (based on the ***POINTS*®** Weight-Loss System) and the Core Plan (focusing on foods with a low energy density) from Weight Watchers provide each of you with your preferred approach. To learn more, go to www.WeightWatchers.com.

Wrapping Things Up

While interest in losing weight is high in both women and men, how they go about pursuing that interest and attempting to lose weight is quite different.

- Women often have more weight-loss experience than men. However, younger men under the age of forty-five are catching up.

- When making the decision to lose weight, women often don't feel as confident as guys do about their potential for success. To boost their confidence, many women spend a great deal of time discussing their options with other people, particularly people who have successfully taken off excess pounds. On the other hand, most men quietly mull over in private the decisions involved in weight loss. If they feel that they need some advice, they are likely to seek it from someone they view as an expert.

- The approaches women and men prefer to use in order to lose weight tend to be different. Women typically spend a great deal of time researching weight-loss options. Because they like to know all the details before they invest their time, women are often attracted to weight-loss approaches that are structured, thorough, and detail-oriented. In contrast, men often prefer approaches that are less time-consuming and less factual. They want to know the bottom line before they get started, yet when men commit themselves to losing weight, they tend to be more compliant and stick to the details of the approach more closely than women do.

Let's Talk!

So you think that it's time to lose weight. Before selecting an approach to try, discuss these questions to help you select the best weight-loss option:

1. What type of weight-loss approaches have you tried in the past and what was your experience with them?

2. How serious are you about losing weight?

3. Do I need to follow the same weight-loss approach as the people I live with?

CHAPTER 8

Women and Men Need to Eat Fewer Calories

What Works and What Doesn't

Department budgets for the next fiscal year are due tomorrow by 5:00 P.M. Coworkers Don and Kay have been working diligently all morning to compile their facts and figures. Long overdue for a lunch break, they agree to walk to the corner deli for a quick bite. Kay's cell phone rings as they walk in the door. She sees that it's her daughter's day care center, so she takes the call and gestures for Don to go ahead and order.

Don, who's thirty-eight, has been trying for the past few weeks to get in shape for a 10K race next month. He's been running every other day, but he noticed that he's not as fast as he was the year before, and he attributes the difference to the spare tire that he seems to have acquired around his middle. So Don has decided to watch what he eats and cut back on some of the high-fat foods he loves, like french fries and burgers. He orders a turkey sandwich on whole-wheat bread with lettuce, tomato, red onion, and mustard (hold the mayo), a bowl of vegetable soup, and a diet soft drink.

Finished with her call, Kay, who's thirty, is starving. She recently returned from maternity leave and is struggling to lose the 40-plus pounds that she gained while pregnant. Stressed out from the call, which brought the news that her baby might be coming down with a cold, she reminds herself not to let her emotions lead her to overeat. So she quickly scans the menu and orders a small chef's salad with fat-free dressing (hold the croutons), a low-fat blueberry muffin, and a 16-ounce bottle of water.

After finding a booth away from the crowd, they sit down and begin to eat.

He says, "How can you eat all of that fat-free stuff? Doesn't it taste like air? It never fills me up. A diet soft drink is the only diet food I can stand."

She says, "I love fat-free foods! They have a lot fewer calories, and they satisfy my cravings for sweets. I like diet soft drinks, too, but I didn't order one because I've heard that drinking water makes you lose weight faster."

Two colleagues grabbing a quick lunch together and then getting back to work: although they don't come out and say it, they are both trying to lose weight. Based on what each of them has ordered, we can conclude that each appears to be making food choices with weight loss in mind. But whose lunch do you think is the better choice? The answer: it may well depend on your gender. Men tend to go for lunches like Don's: other than the diet soft drink, when guys are trying to cut calories, they go for traditional foods to help them feel full and they skip the fat-free stuff. Women, on the other hand, are more likely to have a lunch like Kay's: they're more likely to prefer salads and rely on fat-free dressings, low-fat bakery products, and other calorie-reduced foods as a means of losing weight. And even though water is a healthful beverage, many women mistakenly believe that it is a short cut to weight loss.

The truth of the matter is that men and women alike can lose weight only if they consume fewer calories than they burn. That translates into making changes in one's eating habits. While the majority of women recognize and embrace that fact, guys are apt to resist a bit because men are more likely to believe that they can simply exercise their pounds away. (See chapter 9.) This chapter explores the different beliefs and attitudes that women and men have about eating, cutting back on eating, and the role of food in weight loss.

Foods Men and Women Choose to Help Them Lose

What is the primary reason for America's soaring obesity rates? According to the United States Department of Agriculture (USDA) Economic Research Service, women and men are eating too many calories. The USDA is not alone in that opinion. Data from four National Health and Nutrition Examination Surveys (NHANES) indicate that compared with thirty years ago, men reported consuming an extra 168 calories per day and women an extra 335 calories. While that might not seem like much, it adds up to a lot of extra pounds. Where are the extra calories coming from? According to the USDA, they're from foods laden with sugar and fat: sweetened soft drinks, fried snack foods, fast food, rich pastries, and the like. It stands to reason that if those are the foods that are adding fat to our waistlines, cutting back on them—or their calorie-laden ingredients—is key to losing weight.

To their credit, many women and men are working to reduce the amount of sugar and fat they are eating. But the strategies the genders use to accomplish that tend to vary. It seems that the strategies that men and women prefer to reduce sugar intake are similar, but when it comes to getting fat out of the diet, they choose different paths.

In terms of cutting back on sugar, Weight Watchers research has found that women are more likely than men to cut out sweets like desserts and candy. The same research found that the use of sugar-free products is about the same between the sexes. By far, diet soft drinks are the most frequently consumed sugar-free products. There was a time when your typical guy would not be caught dead drinking a diet cola, weight problem or no weight problem. Those days are gone, however. In today's world, sugar-free soft drinks are now the beverage of choice for a lot of guys, and there is no stigma attached to them, weight problem or no weight problem.

When it comes to fat, reducing saturated fat is an important strategy for everyone working toward losing weight in a healthy way. How that is accomplished, however, tends to differ by gender. Weight Watchers research has found that women are much more likely than men to use fat-free or reduced-fat food products (fat-free salad dressings, low-fat snack chips, reduced-fat ice cream, and so on). Men are more likely to shun such foods, sometimes seeing them as fake or tasting bad. Instead, men rely on more traditional strategies to get fat out of their diets. For example, they continue to use full-fat condiments like mayonnaise, butter, and salad dressing but cut back on the amount; eat fewer fried foods; and find a replacement that naturally contains less fat.

How does that translate into food choices? For example, while a woman will spread low-fat mayonnaise on her sandwich, a man is more inclined to substitute mustard. Or a woman will put a hefty portion of fat-free creamy Italian dressing on her salad, whereas a guy will have a smaller amount of regular creamy Italian dressing or go with an Italian vinaigrette instead.

While both the male and the female strategies can work to reduce calories, is there any evidence that some strategies work better than others when it comes to losing weight? Certainly the switch to sugar-free beverages is a good thing. A 12-ounce can of a sweetened soft drink has at least 12 teaspoons of sugar and no nutrients. When it

Food Swaps to Reduce Fat

Instead of	More women will choose	And more men will choose
coffee with cream	coffee with fat-free creamer	black coffee
a donut	a fat-free bran muffin	a bowl of bran cereal with skim milk
potato chips	fat-free or baked chips	pretzels
bread	2 slices of low-calorie bread	1 slice of whole wheat bread
salami	reduced-fat salami	turkey or ham
cheese	low-fat or reduced-fat cheese	nothing—there is no substitute!
cookies	3 fat-free cookies	a regular cookie, but just one

comes to cutting fat, it appears that the guys' method has a slight edge over the ladies' method. While the ongoing NHANES have determined that both women and men are getting the majority of their extra calories from carbohydrates, only women seem to be picking up extra calories from fat. The average woman's total daily fat intake has increased by 6.5 grams, whereas the average man's has actually decreased by 5.3 grams.

How is it that women can be using so many reduced-fat products and still be consuming more total fat? For starters, many of the reduced-fat food products still provide fat, and if a large portion is eaten, the grams of fat can quickly add up. In addition, relying on reduced-fat foods as a sole strategy for cutting calories from fat can create a false sense of confidence, so that care and awareness when eating foods naturally high in fat—like french fries or burgers—is low. In the long run, some women may be better off eating fewer fat-reduced food products and relying more on some of the men's fat-reduction strategies.

FROM A WOMAN'S VIEWPOINT
FOODS MEN AND WOMEN CHOOSE TO HELP THEM LOSE

Starting a meal with a salad can help both women and men to eat less. Researchers at Penn State University found that people who ate a salad before lunch consumed anywhere from 7 to 12 percent fewer calories at that meal than diners who didn't begin their meal with a salad. But there is a catch: the salad can't be drowning in dressing. While many women avoid the dilemma by opting for a fat-free dressing, that may not be the healthiest option. Studies have also found that people who eat salads topped with fat-free dressings absorb fewer disease-fighting phytonutrients than people who eat their greens with regular dressing. Why? Our bodies need a small amount of fat to absorb certain nutrients. So for the lightest and healthiest salad, use reduced-fat dressings or simply drizzle on a smaller amount of regular dressing.

FROM A MAN'S VIEWPOINT
FOODS MEN AND WOMEN CHOOSE TO HELP THEM LOSE

Not in the mood for a salad, especially if it means eating it with reduced-fat dressing? Then try the soup instead. Several studies have found that eating a bowl of soup reduces feelings of hunger, helps you feel full, and can lower your calorie intake not only for that meal but for the whole day. But not just any soup will do. The most effective are broth-based soups loaded with vegetables and lean meat. So feel free to skip the salad and order soup. And spread the word so women can reap the hunger-satisfying benefits of soup, too.

REAL-LIFE LESSON
Slurping Up the Calories

Situation: My wife and I are trying to lose weight. We have decided to cut out sweetened soft drinks. Rather than switch to diet colas, I'm now drinking a lot of decaffeinated coffee (with just a little sugar and cream), fruit juice, energy drinks, and flavored waters. I'm drinking a lot more beverages now than I used to as a way to avoid eating between meals. The weight is not coming off as quickly as I think it should, and I'm wondering if my choice of beverages has anything to do with it. Any recommendations?

Strategies: It would appear that rather than reduce your caloric intake by eliminating regular soft drinks, you are choosing alternative beverages that also contain calories. And by drinking more beverages throughout the day, the number of calories you're drinking (as opposed to eating) is probably quite high. While the decaffeinated coffee that you're drinking is calorie-free, the sugar and cream you are adding are not. Fruit juice can provide a lot of calories. Likewise, most energy drinks contain a fair number of calories, as do flavored waters. You need to read the labels of these products carefully to make sure that your choices are not laden with calories. There is one other factor that you'll want to keep in mind in your beverage selection. It appears people's bodies do not "recognize" the calories consumed in beverages in the same way that they do food. That means you can drink a lot of calories without your body sending out an "I feel full" signal to the brain. While your strategy to use beverages to avoid eating between meals is a good one, it will work only if the beverages you choose aren't full of calories. One way to keep the strategy and keep it simple is to stick to tap or bottled water.

Eating Strategies: What Does and Doesn't Work

Women and men approach the concept of calories in and calories out from very different vantage points. Whereas women usually go right to the calories in (eating less), men are more likely to head for the calories out (working out more). When it comes to losing weight, the female approach has the definite advantage. As mentioned, it's virtually impossible to lose a sizeable amount of weight with exercise alone. (See chapter 9 for more details.) So when guys are serious about losing weight, finding strategies that will help them reduce their calories is a must.

When it comes to eating strategies, there are some innate differences between the sexes. Based on research conducted for Weight Watchers, we conclude that women tend to use a wide variety of detail-oriented tactics, including decreasing portion sizes, counting calories, following a structured eating plan, eating more fruits and vegetables, and keeping a food diary. As we saw in chapter 7, women tend to be more bottom-up thinkers, which means that they are drawn to putting together several small tactics to create an overall eating strategy for weight loss.

Although many men can and do lose weight using such tactics, some men, particularly guys with less than 40 pounds to lose, often find them too restrictive and too complicated. They prefer limiting the number of tactics to the few that will do the most good.

While many of the eating strategies that women use to lose weight are effective, others have limited value as stand-alone methods. For example, women are far more likely than men to use meal replacements or shakes or to take medication to shed extra pounds. Although some of these strategies may be helpful tools, they are unlikely to lead to lasting weight loss without being part of a broader lifestyle modification effort.

In addition, many women believe that drinking large amounts of water is critical to losing weight. Although drinking water is certainly a good thing to do for your overall health, there is scant scientific evidence to back up the claim that it helps weight loss. In fact, studies have found that drinking water before, during, and after a meal makes no significant difference in the amount of food eaten.

Women and men do have some favorite strategies in their pursuit of weight loss, but they're not particularly helpful. Both genders gravitate toward eating strategies that provide only a temporary fix and set them up for future weight regain. The first is skipping meals as a means of cutting back their overall food consumption. This strategy often backfires because eventually the dieter becomes so hungry that he or she overeats. And if the skipped meal is breakfast, it may be an even bigger mistake. According to the National Weight Control Registry, eating breakfast every day is one of the strategies associated with lasting weight loss.

A second failed strategy is completely eliminating certain foods, like chocolate or potato chips, because they are hard to resist. While that strategy can be effective in the early days of weight loss, as weight loss progresses, the effectiveness wanes. In fact, most people find themselves desiring the forbidden food to the point that when it is finally eaten, what's eaten is a supersized portion. Rather than deciding to eliminate certain foods forever, a more effective strategy is to learn how to include them periodically in an overall eating strategy that supports weight loss.

A third approach with questionable effectiveness is becoming a vegetarian. Although it can be a healthy eating alternative, simply avoiding meat and animal products doesn't guarantee weight loss—candy, cookies, and many snack foods are all vegetarian choices.

Finally, it seems as though every other decade, many women and men try to follow a very-high-protein diet to lose weight. Thankfully, people have come to realize that such a diet does not work in the long term.

Looking at the more positive side, men and women do share some safe and effective eating strategies that can help them eat less food and lose weight. As we discussed, both women and men prefer to reduce their sugar and fat intake as a strategy for cutting back. In addition, Weight Watchers research has found that women and men are equally likely to try to reduce their between-meal snacking. That is a good thing, given that snacking is on the rise in the United States. According to the USDA's nationally representative surveys, snacks now account for up to 25 percent of our daily energy intake, which many health professionals think may account for the extra calories that all Americans, including kids, are consuming. Also, in a study by Weight Watchers, both women and men said that they were cutting back on alcohol. Again, that is another excellent tactic, given that alcoholic beverages provide a generous number of empty calories. In addition, people who drink alcohol are often more vulnerable to letting down their guard and may find themselves overeating in social situations—at a party, in a restaurant, or at a ball game.

Basically, both women and men seem to have some unique preferences for eating strategies that can help them cut back. Women frequently opt for a more structured eating plan, whereas men often do better when they cut back on their snacking and drink less alcohol. The bottom line: one size doesn't fit all.

FROM A WOMAN'S VIEWPOINT
EATING STRATEGIES: WHAT DOES AND DOESN'T WORK

Portion sizes have exploded for just about all foods and food categories—desserts, salty snacks, soft drinks, bagels, french fries, and burgers. Portion sizes for many popular foods and beverages are two to five times larger than they were when those foods were first introduced. So how do women respond to supersizing? Since women are more likely than men to cut calories by eating smaller portions, they prefer to downsize. Many women have no problem ordering a small skim latte, eating half a bagel, or sharing their husband's dessert (a lot of guys hate when a woman asks the waiter for an extra fork!).

FROM A MAN'S VIEWPOINT
EATING STRATEGIES: WHAT DOES AND DOESN'T WORK

Men generally have no problem with giant-size portions. What guy can resist the all-you-can-eat buffet? But men might want to rethink their eating strategies, especially if they are trying to cut back. Several studies have found that the larger the portion that is served, the more people eat—sometimes up to 26 percent more. So rather than take an approach that works for women (downsizing), guys might be better off trying to find ways to bulk up their meals without adding many calories. Examples include adding lots of low-calorie extras to their sandwich or burrito, such as lettuce, tomato, and onion; ordering a thin-crust pizza with extra veggies; or adding chopped fruits or berries to their cereal.

REAL-LIFE LESSON
Eating on the Road

Situation: I'm a forty-five-year-old salesman. My job keeps me on the road about 75 percent of the time, so I live my life on airplanes and in hotel rooms with minibars. I also eat most of my meals in restaurants, often entertaining clients. Can you give me some tips on how to lose weight given my lifestyle?

Strategies: Being a road warrior can play havoc on the waistline. It's especially difficult when you're playing host to clients and need to set the example for an indulgent meal. Here are a few tips that may help. First, order a light and healthy breakfast, like a poached egg on whole wheat toast with fruit or bran flakes and skim milk. Getting your day off to a good start without a lot of calories can help you as your day progresses. Second, do not accept the key to the minibar when you check into the hotel. That will help you avoid the can of cashews when the late-night munchies hit. When entertaining clients, rely on low-calorie starters to fill you up at the start. Good choices are shrimp cocktail, broth-based soup, mixed green salad, or oysters on the half shell. Select entrées that are simple and grilled—sirloin steak, pork chops, or salmon—and skip the sauces. If you're ordering wine, keep the bottle near you so that you can top off your client's glasses but keep from filling your own. For dessert, order a coffee or cappuccino to enjoy while your guests are having something else. Finally, prepare yourself for long plane rides by bringing lower-calorie choices on board with you. That helps you avoid the higher-calorie snack foods that many airlines offer and keeps you from getting off the plane famished and therefore tempted to overeat as soon as you get settled. By recognizing the challenges of living on the road and having plans in place to deal with them as they arise, you can successfully lose weight.

The Emotional Impact of Eating Less

Reducing the calories they consume is the only way men and women can lose weight. But anybody who's ever tried to shed a few pounds knows it's easier said than done. Despite the fact that there are so many excellent strategies women and men can use to help themselves and each other scale back their eating, emotions can get in the way. How women and men think and feel ultimately affects their eating behavior. And the reality is that even under the same circumstances, women and men often have very different emotional responses to eating, and those responses can cause them to overeat rather than cut back.

Take food cravings, for example. Even though men don't necessarily refer to them as cravings (see chapter 4), just about everyone who is trying to eat less and lose weight experiences them to some extent.

Bruce and Nancy Rogers and their daughter, Catherine
ONTARIO, CANADA

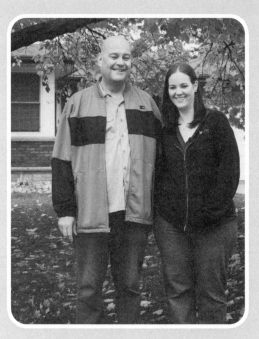

Bruce and Catherine Rogers

About ten years ago, Bruce suffered from two heart attacks and was diagnosed with type 2 diabetes—and he was only forty-six years old. He says, "My doctor told me to lose weight or make sure that my estate was in order." At 6 feet 3 inches and 305 pounds, Bruce had never been heavier and was not sure what to do. The doctor prescribed a diabetic diet, and that worked for a while, but Bruce's job, working as an investigator for the Canadian customs bureau, kept him busy, and he felt that the diet was too complicated and too inconvenient. So for help he turned to his wife, Nancy, who works as a lab technologist at the local hospital. Nancy, who is just over 5 feet 8 inches and weighed 249 pounds, had been struggling with her weight too. She says, "I researched every book, program, and medication out there. We tried so many, but none of them really worked." She had some success on a very-low-calorie diet, losing about 80 pounds, but she says, "My energy level was so low and I felt tired and sick most of the time, so I stopped the diet and quickly gained back all the weight."

Catherine, their twenty-five-year-old daughter who lives with them, had weight problems of her own. She explains, "I was fed up with how I looked, and my dad's heart problems and diabetes really scared me." Catherine is 5 feet 7 inches and weighed about 290 pounds. She'd made several attempts to lose weight on her own but never lost more than 10 pounds and felt constantly deprived.

After ten years of trying to lose weight, Bruce, Nancy, and Catherine were all ready to give up. Then Nancy discovered Weight Watchers. "My best friend's father lost 160 pounds on the program. He was so convinced that the program worked that he even became a leader." So all three of them joined at the same time, and all three are now successfully losing weight using the Flex Plan. Bruce likes the flexibility of Weight Watchers and so far has lost about 51 pounds. He says, "I've always been a grazer, snacking all day long, usually on something salty and crunchy." Now he's eating regularly scheduled meals, lots of fruits and vegetables, and more grilled foods (he threw away the family's deep fryer!), and to satisfy his desire for crunchy snacks he buys single-serving bags of microwave popcorn. A few months after starting Weight Watchers, he started swimming a few times a week.

Nancy loves the Weight Watchers program, too, and has lost around 29 pounds. She says, "During the week we don't eat out as much as we used to. I try to buy the light frozen dinners for all of us so that we can have something quick." Nancy thinks the Flex Plan is simple and easy to follow. She says, "I've had a lot of fun teaching Bruce how to read the food labels when we do our weekly shopping. He wasn't that interested at first. Now he's the one telling me which foods to buy!" Nancy confesses that sweets are still her weakness. She says, "I buy reduced-fat ice cream and low-fat cookies, which seem to do the trick." She also likes to use products like fat-free salad dressings and low-calorie bread.

Of the three of them, Catherine has been the most successful with Weight Watchers so far. She's lost over 75 pounds and is having a great deal of fun shopping for new clothes. She says, "I went from size 2X pants to ladies large. I look so different that a friend who had not seen me in a while didn't even recognize me when we got together!" Catherine has learned to enjoy her new way of eating, and when she does get a craving for chocolate, she chooses a piece of chocolate with a low **POINTS**® value instead of a candy bar.

All three family members agree that Weight Watchers is not a diet; it's a healthy way of eating for the rest of your life. They all felt that participating together has been the best thing of all. Catherine says, "We all try to look out for one another. One of our favorite lines is 'Keep it up and keep it off.' We are all still actively in the process of losing weight." According to Nancy, "With Weight Watchers, there is no such thing as deprivation. You just have to remind yourself to think before you eat."

Weight Watchers research has confirmed that men are just as likely as women to report getting food cravings while on a weight-loss diet. Yet how women and men respond to a food craving tends to be very different—and based on their emotions. Women tend to overeat when they feel down or depressed, whereas men tend to overeat when they feel happy.

According to a study conducted by researchers at McGill University in Canada, women and men reach for different foods to satisfy their cravings. Women indulge in foods like candy and cookies to try to feel better or improve their mood. Men, on the other hand, get cravings for food when they're already in a good mood. So to keep their spirits high, guys are more likely to indulge in high-protein comfort foods, like a 16-ounce thick, juicy steak. In addition to finding that women and men satisfy their cravings with different foods, the study found that only the women reported feeling guilty about eating in response to a craving. Why? Women may be more tuned into the fact that they are overeating and choosing foods that have a lot of calories. Given that they're trying to lose weight, they may be quicker to realize what they've done and more vulnerable to feelings of guilt.

Social situations are another example of how gender plays into the emotional elements of eating. Compared with men, women spend more time thinking about their weight and have a tendency to be concerned with other people's opinions of it (see chapter 3). When a woman finds herself in a social situation that is centered on food—an office party or a holiday gathering, for example—she can go into the situation thinking "Danger! Be on full alert"—she knows that food will be everywhere and that the possibility of responding emotionally by overeating is high. If she's feeling good, chances are she'll be able to control her eating. But if she's feeling stressed or insecure, she's more likely to make a beeline for the dessert table and, after overindulging, wind up feeling guilty. Whether a woman resists or gives into the temptation to eat, the bottom line on social eating for women is that they need to be aware of how their emotions influence their eating and be ready with strategies to compensate.

Social situations for men are a different story. According to Weight Watchers research, men are much less likely than women to report overeating in response to being in a negative emotional state. Rather, men say that the major reason for overeating is being in a social situation (such as a picnic or BBQ) where an abundance of food is readily available. The research also revealed that men were more likely than women to overeat after drinking. What's important to keep in mind is that even though men recognized that social situations triggered them to overeat, they were unable to make the connection between being in a positive emotional state and overeating. So when guys attend social events, they are often caught off guard and are more likely than women to overindulge.

It appears that guys need to borrow a page from the ladies' emotional-eating strategy book. When men are trying to lose weight and cut back on their food intake, they need to go on the offensive and be aware of their emotional eating so that they can set up a winning weight-loss defense.

FROM A WOMAN'S VIEWPOINT
THE EMOTIONAL IMPACT OF EATING LESS

PMS, bad news from the boss, a parking ticket—many women eat when they feel down and are likely to turn to food to pick up their mood. But they have also developed strategies that help them resist their emotional eating. Many women use the avoidance tactic—no ice cream or chocolate in the house, no walking past the bakery on the way home from work. But women's favorite strategy is the emotional rescue—talking about their problem with friends and family members. Talking things out often helps them feel better and, at the very least, helps them figure out ways to curtail their impulses to eat in response to emotions.

FROM A MAN'S VIEWPOINT
THE EMOTIONAL IMPACT OF EATING LESS

While most men tend to be less aware of their emotional overeating and how it affects their weight loss, some men appear to be more attuned to their emotions. A study conducted by researchers in the Netherlands discovered that obese men with a BMI over 38 appeared to be very aware of their tendency to eat emotionally, although the men found it difficult to identify or explain the feelings responsible for their overeating. It looks as if some guys do know that they are emotional eaters; they just need help learning how to express it.

REAL-LIFE LESSON
Eating after 8:00 P.M.

Situation: I'm very concerned about my husband's health. He has terrible arthritis, and his doctor has said that if he doesn't lose some weight he may need a hip replacement. We have both been trying to eat less and have lost some weight—he's lost even more than I have! But he just started a new job and is now working the night shift. I have heard that if you eat after 8:00 P.M., you'll gain weight. Is that true? I would hate to see him gain back all the weight he's lost.

Strategies: The idea that nighttime eating leads to weight gain is common. The truth is that the time of day at which calories are consumed doesn't matter, so the notion that food eaten at night turns to fat quicker than food eaten during the day is false. For many people, nighttime eating is associated with mindless snacking. Those nighttime calories add up quickly and lead to weight gain. The trick for your husband is to schedule his eating in a way that fits his job and is normal. That may mean having dinner with you, then "lunch" at work at 2:00 A.M., and breakfast before going to bed when he gets home from work. His day then becomes your night, and that means little or no eating (such as joining you for lunch). One more thing that your husband should be on the lookout for is getting enough sleep. It is not uncommon for night-shift workers to have erratic sleeping patterns and deprive themselves of much-needed rest. Sleep deprivation can undermine the best-intentioned weight-loss effort. By planning sensible meals on and off the job and getting adequate sleep, you husband should be able to have continued weight-loss success.

Wrapping Things Up

Women and men who are serious about losing weight understand that they have to cut back on the amount of food they eat. Exercise alone isn't enough. But women and men go about doing this in different ways, ways that are unique to their gender.

- In terms of deciding what to cut back on, women and men agree that sugar and fat need to go. Whereas both have no qualms about drinking sugar-free soft drinks as a sugar-reduction strategy, their fat-reduction strategies are not similar. Women frequently rely on fat-free and low-fat foods, such as fat-free salad dressings and low-fat treats, to reduce fat; men are less apt to enjoy eating those products. Guys use a more effective strategy—they eat foods that naturally have less fat, like turkey or lean ham; they use less butter; and they stop eating fried foods. Overall, the guys' approach tends to cut more calories than the women's approach.

- Women and men seem to have different preferences for eating strategies that will enable them to cut back, but they do agree on one thing: the strategy needs to result in long-term weight loss and be one that they can follow for the rest of their lives. Women tend to enjoy more structured weight-loss plans, plans that involve counting, reducing, and record-keeping. Although some men are willing to follow those types of plans—and often do better on them than the women—many guys prefer a different kind of structure. An eating plan that's attractive to guys often involves few details— a "tell me what I can and can't eat" approach—and provides for generous portions. The reality for both women and men when choosing a weight-loss plan is that as long as it's well-balanced and safe, the format and structure are really up to the person following the plan.

- Emotions can make or break weight-loss success, and although it may come as a surprise to some men, both women and men are emotional eaters. The emotions that trigger the eating are just different. Women have a tendency to overeat when they get the blues; men tend to overeat when they are feeling good. Emotional eating is a weight-loss area in which women seem to have the advantage. Since women are more aware than guys of the tendencies to eat emotionally, they may be more proactive in dealing with them. Unlike most guys, most women talk about their emotional eating, a strategy that often helps them feel better and find solutions.

Let's Talk!

So you're both interested in losing weight, and you're committed to eating less. But before you select a program to follow, be sure to take inventory of what each of you is willing to do in the long term. Here are some questions to help you narrow your options:

1. Which foods that contain a lot of sugar and/or fat do you enjoy? How will you deal with them once you commit yourself to losing weight?

2. What strategies have you used in the past to lose weight? What did you like about them? What didn't you like about them?

3. What situations seem to trigger your overeating? How do you feel before and after you overeat? What can you do to change the situation or the way you react to it?

CHAPTER 9

Move More to Keep It Off

Neighbors Marianne and Chris belong to the same health club. Chris is forty-three years old, married, and the father of three kids. Last winter he tore a ligament in his knee playing basketball with his buddies. While convalescing, he put on about 15 pounds. He attributes the gain to the fact that he couldn't exercise and he never changed his eating habits—he continued drinking a few beers at night while munching on nuts and chips. Now that his doctor has told him he can resume his former level of activity, Chris has been going to his club at least four times a week. He spends most of the time lifting weights and using the new elliptical trainer that's equipped with heart-rate monitors and variable-incline settings. Even though Chris attends the club regularly, he's been able to drop only a few pounds over the past several months.

Marianne, forty-one years old, is a good friend of Chris's. Marianne went through a painful divorce about a year ago and has put on 25 pounds. She blames the gain on her new late-night love affair with chocolate chip ice cream and the fact that she's working long hours and has little time to exercise. To help shed some of the excess pounds, she's been watching what she eats, cutting back on the ice cream, eating more fruits and vegetables, and trimming her portion sizes. So far Marianne has lost about 10 pounds over the past 3 months, but she feels her progress has been too slow.

As Chris is leaving the weight room, he bumps into Marianne, who is coming out of a step class. They exchange greetings. Chris mentions that he hasn't seen Marianne at the club before, and they get into a discussion about their weight-loss efforts.

He says, "When I first started exercising, I lost some weight, but now I'm at a standstill. I think I need to up the intensity of my training sessions."

Marianne agrees that exercise is important but confesses that she comes to the club only sporadically. She says, "I really want to work out more, but I have to travel constantly for my job, so when I'm home, I want to be with the kids—I feel guilty coming here! I've been on a diet, but I think I'm going to have to try something else, like fasting, to speed up the weight loss."

Exercise does play an important role in weight loss, but exercise alone, without limiting calories from food, is not enough to promote a sizeable weight loss. Research has shown that it is virtually impossible to lose weight taking the exercise-only route. Unfortunately, people are generally unaware of that fact, particularly men. When guys like Chris first attempt to shed excess pounds, they often place too much emphasis on exercise and overlook or underestimate the value of cutting back on their calories. Women typically approach weight loss more like Marianne: they don't rely on exercise as their main strategy for slimming down but focus more on what and how much they're eating, an approach that is definitely to their advantage (see chapter 8). However, women like Marianne often have unrealistic expectations about their weight loss. All too often they become impatient with the rate at which the pounds are coming off, especially if they compare themselves with men, who are physically equipped to lose weight more quickly. So instead of trying to exercise more, women have a tendency to look for other diet-related approaches to cut calories even faster, and that isn't a healthy or practical strategy. Unfortunately, that unrealistic approach can set women up for disappointment and lead them to abandon their commitment to losing weight.

The best way for women and men to lose weight is for them to narrow the gender gap and combine their strategies. As the example of Chris and Marianne illustrates, women and men have different attitudes and beliefs about the role physical activity plays in weight loss. In this chapter we explore those differences to help everyone come up with a winning weight-loss strategy.

Why Exercise Alone Doesn't Work

It's a fact: based on the pool of scientific evidence, health and medical experts agree that while exercise is important, it does not lead to significant weight loss on its own. As we saw in chapter 5, although it *is* theoretically possible to lose weight using exercise as one's sole weight-loss strategy, that approach is not realistic for most people. The reality for both men and women is that without paying careful attention, it is very easy to eat the calories burned in exercise. For example, it takes about 1 hour on the treadmill for a man of 170 pounds to burn off a bagel (without cream cheese), a few cookies, or a donut. Each 30-minute session that a woman spends circuit training burns about 150 calories. For a 150-pound woman, that's the equivalent of a 12-ounce glass of orange juice. Still not convinced? Here are some other examples that illustrate how long women and men need to exercise (at moderate intensity) to burn off some of their favorite indulgence foods.

If a 170-pound man ate or drank	*He would have to spend*
2 pieces of deep-dish pepperoni pizza	2½ hours walking briskly
a 12-ounce bottle of beer	45 minutes raking leaves
a ½-cup handful of peanuts	1¾ hours washing the car
a 5-ounce serving of nachos with cheese	1¾ hours bicycling on flat terrain
a 12-ounce broiled steak	2¼ hours swimming
If a 150-pound woman ate or drank	*She would have to spend*
A 16-ounce coffee mocha without whipped cream	1½ hours walking briskly
1 fudge-walnut brownie	1¾ hours vacuuming
1 cup of butter pecan ice cream	1½ hours doing aerobic dancing
a 4-ounce glass of white wine	½ hour doing yoga
1 slice chocolate chip cheesecake	1½ hours lifting weights

Another factor to consider on the subject of why exercise alone doesn't seem to help most people lose much weight has to do with the power of estimation: people have trouble determining their eating and exercise levels accurately. Research has found that it is very common to underestimate the number of calories consumed in food. At the same time, numerous studies have found that it is also very common to overestimate the time spent engaged in activity. For example, a University of Pittsburgh School of Medicine study followed fifty overweight women involved in a behavioral weight control program. Participants were required to exercise for 30 minutes. One group exercised for 30 minutes without a break; the other group exercised in three 10-minute spurts. All of the women were asked to record their activity in a daily exercise log. To validate their self-reported information, they wore a device that measured their activity. The results? Approximately 45 percent of the women overreported the amount of exercise they performed, and there was no difference between the women engaged in long bouts of exercise and those engaged in short bouts. Even more alarming: the women who overreported their exercise lost on average 3 pounds less than the women who underreported their exercise. While this study was done with women, the same results would likely be seen in men.

A more effective and more realistic approach than exercising alone is to split the caloric difference. Begin by reducing calories from food and then add exercise to your strategy.

FROM A WOMAN'S VIEWPOINT
WHY EXERCISE ALONE DOESN'T WORK

Women are notorious for believing that their metabolism is out of whack. Based on over ten years of research, however, researchers have concluded that women may want to reconsider that statement. A classic study conducted in 1992 concluded that not shedding pounds can rarely be attributed to a malfunction of the thyroid, the metabolism, or any other body function. People in the study were not losing weight mainly because they had inaccurate perceptions of what they ate and how much they exercised. On average, they underreported how much they ate by 47 percent and overreported how much they exercised by 51 percent. One potential solution to this dilemma: Keep a daily journal.

FROM A MAN'S VIEWPOINT
WHY EXERCISE ALONE DOESN'T WORK

What can you expect from an eat-less-and-exercise combination? According to a 2004 study performed in Australia, a lot. Researchers assigned sixty nonsmoking overweight men between the ages of twenty and fifty to four groups: one was on a reduced-calorie diet and engaged in light exercise three times per week; a second was on a reduced-calorie diet and engaged in vigorous exercise three times per week; the third engaged in light exercise only; and the fourth engaged in vigorous exercise only. The men who restricted their eating and exercised three times a week for 16 weeks lost an average of 22 pounds and showed improvements in their blood sugar and insulin levels, whereas those in the exercise-only groups lost only 1 to 3 pounds. Interestingly, the weight-loss difference between the light and vigorous exercise groups was only a couple of pounds. The men in the vigorous exercise groups experienced improvement in their blood sugar levels, with the effect being greater when the exercise was coupled with the reduced-calorie diet.

Coming to Terms with Physical Activity

Need some help translating the exercise lingo? Here's what some of the key terms really mean:

moderate intensity physical activity: A person exercising at this level should experience some increase in his or her breathing or heart rate. While working out at a moderate intensity level, it's fairly easy to carry on a conversation. Moderate-intensity activities include walking briskly, mowing the lawn, dancing, swimming, and bicycling on level terrain.

vigorous intensity physical activity: A person exercising at this level should experience a large increase in breathing or heart rate. Conversation while working out is difficult or broken. Examples of vigorous-intensity exercise are jogging, mowing the lawn with a push mower, high-impact aerobic dancing, swimming continuous laps, bicycling uphill, and carrying more than 25 pounds up a flight of stairs.

regular physical activity: Physical activity is considered regular if it is performed most days of the week, preferably daily; five or more times for moderate-intensity activities, three or more times for vigorous intensity activities.

REAL-LIFE LESSON
Weight-Conscious Workout Options

Situation: I'm a thirty-year-old single woman and I'm very over-weight. My doctor told me that I have at least 100 pounds to lose. I've started reducing my portions and eating more fruits and vegeta-bles and so far I've lost 40 pounds. I know that working out would help me lose even more weight. My friends keep trying to get me to come with them to their health club, but they are all so skinny! I am too embarrassed to go there. Can you recommend some exer-cises for people who are overweight and self-conscious?

Strategies: Congratulations! You've already lost a large amount of weight. And it is great that you are considering adding exercise to your calorie-cutting efforts. Not only will adding exercise enhance your weight loss now, but once you've lost the weight, exercise will also be one of the key things you can do to keep the pounds off forever.

If you are not ready to join your friends at their health club, you may want to consider walking. Walking is by far the most popular activity among those working to lose weight, and it's not by chance. Walking doesn't require athletic skill, special equipment, or a gym membership, and it has a low risk of injury. In addition, walking can be done alone or with others—the option is up to you. You need only buy a good pair of walking shoes—an investment well worth the money—and go! Walking is also a year-round activity. You can walk outside when the weather is cooperating, move to an indoor facility like a shopping mall when the weather is uncooperative, or buy a treadmill if you prefer to watch television while covering the miles.

Although walking is a great exercise for most people, it may not be your cup of tea, and when it comes to exercise, doing something you enjoy is the single most important factor. With that in mind, other options that may appeal to you or come in handy if you get bored with walking are working out to exercise videos or DVDs, which you can do at home or doing water aerobics, a great form of exercise that is especially helpful to people with physical limitations.

Exercise: A Matter of Priority

Overall, women and men seem to have very different views on how exercise best fits into the weight-loss equation. Several studies have found that men prioritize exercise first and food second; women prioritize food first and exercise second.

Why do men have a tendency to start with exercise when they need to shed some pounds? One logical answer is that many men have more experience with exercise, going back to their boyhoods. In addition, men who exercise regularly often see physical results. The majority of men typically gain weight in their midsection or stomach (taking on what is commonly referred to as the apple shape), a fat-deposit area that puts them at increased risk for certain diseases, such as heart disease and diabetes (see chapter 2). Studies have shown that regular exercise has a strong effect on reducing waist circumference in men, and that in turn helps reduce their disease risk. So when guys are suddenly able to buckle their belt a notch or two tighter or fit into a smaller-size pair of pants, they see the effects of exercise and are likely to discount the impact of eating less.

Although women are definitely on the right weight-loss track when they cut back their calories from food, eventually they will need to add some exercise, especially if they seem to find themselves in a weight-loss rut. That is when most women could use some help from the guys. A 2006 Weight Watchers study discovered that women's awareness of the need for regular exercise is high and even comparable to men's, but awareness is not the same as action. As we saw in chapter 5, women in general tend to be less physically active than men. When women watch the needle on the scale fall, they are more likely to attribute their weight loss to their diet than to exercise, and they are correct in making that assumption. But when women reach a point where their weight loss levels off or stalls, they have a tendency to restrict their calories from food even more rather than adding exercise to their weight-loss regimen.

Since it's next to impossible to lose weight using only exercise, the female eat-less approach is going to be the better strategy and result in greater weight loss—provided that the reduced food intake is done in a healthy and balanced way (see chapter 8). Down the road, though, the male exercise-more approach helps enhance weight loss and will be one of the key strategies for keeping pounds off for good.

FROM A WOMAN'S VIEWPOINT
EXERCISE: A MATTER OF PRIORITY

Weight Watchers conducted research to find out about women's physical activity preferences and discovered that women like to keep their exercise routine simple. Hands down, women enjoyed walking over any other type of exercise. Some other physical activities that women were more likely than men to participate in included lifting weights and taking yoga, Pilates, or kickboxing classes. Women's equipment choices also reflected their desire for simplicity. Just give a woman a gym bag, a yoga mat, a water bottle, and a pair of workout shoes, and she's ready to exercise.

FROM A MAN'S VIEWPOINT
EXERCISE: A MATTER OF PRIORITY

Based on Weight Watchers research, walking also appears to be men's number one choice for exercise, but men prefer to branch out and sweat more. Guys, particularly those under the age of forty-five, were more likely than women and men over the age of forty-five to participate in such sports as tennis, golf, basketball, and cycling. When guys exercise, they typically enjoy all the physical aspects of it: sweating, pumping iron, building muscles. Not only do they enjoy working out, but they are also intrigued by the wide variety of state-of-the-art exercise gadgets out there, such as body-fat scales, pedometers, and heart rate wristwatches, to name just a few. Men often find such gadgets fun and inspirational. Women, on the other hand, are less infatuated with them and often find them unnecessary and overly complicated.

REAL-LIFE LESSON
Eat Less Versus Exercise More: Where to Begin?

Situation: My husband and I have tried to lose weight in the past, but we never took it seriously and gained back any weight that we lost. This time we're going to do it right. We know that if we want to keep the pounds off, we need to change our eating and exercise habits, but taking both on at once is overwhelming. I said that we should focus on our eating habits, but my husband feels it's more important to start exercising first. Any suggestions on how we should get started?

Strategies: That is a terrific question! In general, it is better to treat changing your eating habits and becoming more active as two separate events. Why? Different behavior changes that are begun at the same time are more likely to be abandoned at the same time, but if the changes are made separately and one is discontinued, it will have a minimal impact on the other. When it comes to weight loss, your best bet is to start by reducing food calories. Pick a healthful eating plan and take a few weeks to get comfortable with it. Because a reduction in your food intake has a greater potential to bring about noticeable weight loss than exercise does, a few weeks of reducing your calories should have you both feeling good about your progress. Then, once you feel comfortable with the changes in your eating, start on exercise. By having both changes in place within a month or so of beginning your weight-loss effort, you'll get the advantages of both without being overwhelmed by too much change at the beginning.

COUPLES UP CLOSE

Gary and Dorothy Stice
OKLAHOMA

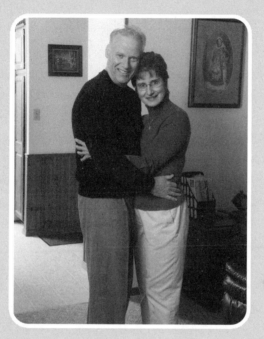

Gary and Dorothy have been married over thirty years. About ten years ago they decided to start their own computer software company, which they operate out of their home. They have both thoroughly enjoyed running the business together, as it has given them tremendous flexibility in their schedules and enabled them to focus on other interests, such as their health. According to Gary, "All of our lives we had always been round-shaped people. Dorothy developed diabetes, and because of my weight, I was suffering from all kinds of health problems—hypertension, high blood cholesterol, and sleep apnea." Dorothy adds, "We were both on many types of medication, and we were not even fifty years old!" Gary's sleep apnea was so severe that he twice had near-fatal car accidents.

The year they both turned fifty, Gary and Dorothy felt that they needed to do something to get healthier. "At age fifty our insurance premiums doubled, and we were fed up with being on medication," says Gary. So that year their birthday presents to each other were Weight Watchers memberships—and losing weight together. In addition to making changes in their meals, they started walking about 2 miles most days of the week. Dorothy agrees. She says, "It was really hard at first to walk because we were both so big and out of shape. But we gradually worked our way up, and now it's just a regular part of our day." Gary lost weight much faster than Dorothy, but she isn't complaining. She says, "It seems as if men can just walk around the block and lose weight. We women need to be aware that we have to work out twice as much to get even a fraction of the weight loss that men get!" Gary agrees that men have a tremendous advantage over women because of their body muscle-to-fat ratios, but he adds, "It seems that women and men have equally tough times keeping the pounds from returning once they've lost weight." In addition to watching what and how much they ate, Dorothy began taking a Pilates class twice a week at a community recreation center. She says, "I just fell in love with it! And I like the fact that I was taking the class with women and men who were my age, not superyoung people wearing spandex!" Dorothy was so taken with Pilates that when the instructor could no longer teach the class due to an injury, Dorothy was eventually able to take over. Gary started spending more time at the community center, too. He began lifting weights and developed a network of friends with whom he enjoys exercising on a regular basis.

After a year and a half, Gary and Dorothy had reached their weight-loss goals. Now they are off all medications and are Weight Watchers lifetime members. Gary's waist went from a size 40 to a 33 and his neck size is down 3 inches. Dorothy's success has been terrific, too. "I've lost about

58 pounds and I never want to find it again!" she says. Both feel that on their own they could have lost the weight successfully, but the pounds would not have come off as quickly and the process wouldn't have been as much fun. Dorothy says, "We think the perfect gift that someone can give the one he or she loves is the gift of making the commitment to getting lighter and healthier as a couple."

Exercise Benefits: Weight Loss and Beyond

If exercise alone does not promote a substantial weight loss, why bother? For starters, when exercise is coupled with a reduced-calorie eating plan, it enhances weight loss. But the area where exercise appears to have its greatest impact is in weight maintenance. Exercise is a key strategy for keeping weight off. In fact, several studies have shown that regular physical activity is one of the best predictors of who will be able to maintain weight loss successfully.

Exercise is essential to preventing lost pounds from reappearing. Most people in the National Weight Control Registry are between the ages of forty-four and forty-nine, and about 20 percent are men. What's fascinating to observe in this group of successful losers is that 89 percent of the participants used diet and physical activity together to lose weight, and 91 percent reported using extensive physical activity to keep the weight off. The average amount of energy they burned with exercise was 2,500 calories per week for women and 3,300 calories per week for men. That is a very high level of physical activity and breaks down to doing about 60 to 90 minutes of moderate-intensity physical activity (such as brisk walking, raking leaves, or bicycling on level ground) per day.

If getting in 60 to 90 minutes of any type of physical activity every day sounds impossible, don't throw in the exercise towel just yet. According to the U.S. Surgeon General's Report on Physical Activity and Health, every little bit of exercise helps. Numerous studies have found that 30 minutes of moderate-intensity physical activity above and beyond one's usual daily physical activity on most if not all days of the week provide a multitude of health benefits, such as a reduced risk of heart disease, high blood pressure, high cholesterol, premature death, colon and breast cancer, and diabetes. It can also improve the health of muscles, bones, and joints. And studies are continuing to find that exercising regularly can reduce stress and improve mental health.

What's even more motivating about the benefits of exercise is that the 30 minutes of physical activity don't have to be done all at once. Physical activity can be accumulated over the course of the day in short bouts. For example, 10 minutes of brisk walking, 10 minutes of light gardening, and 10 minutes of raking leaves add up to 30 minutes of moderate physical activity and you reap the same health benefits as someone who exercised for 30 minutes all at once. Certainly the more anyone exercises, whether moderately or vigorously, the more calories are burned.

The key to exercising is finding activities that are enjoyable. Start with a goal of 30 minutes a day, gradually working up to it by taking a walk after dinner, climbing stairs instead of taking an elevator, or getting up to change the television channel rather than using the remote. Then find ways to increase the time, such as adding 10 minutes to a daily walk, taking an aerobics class, or golfing without a cart and carrying the clubs.

The take-away message is that eventually exercise needs to be part of everyone's weight-management plan, particularly after losing weight, so that the pounds will disappear for good.

FROM A WOMAN'S VIEWPOINT
EXERCISE BENEFITS: WEIGHT LOSS AND BEYOND

When it comes to exercise, women certainly enjoy the physical results they achieve, such as getting more toned and dropping a pants size. But what really motivates many women to participate in regular physical activity is that they also enjoy the way exercise makes them feel. It's not uncommon for a woman to say, "On days I don't exercise, I feel crabby" or "I don't feel good about myself unless I get a walk in every day." Basically, the better a woman feels about exercise, the more likely she is to work out regularly. A study conducted in 2006 found that when overweight women lost weight by following a behavioral weight-loss program (exercise and a diet that moderately restricted calorie intake), those with a weight loss of 10 percent or more reported feeling more confident about exercising and exercised more compared with women who engaged in lower levels of physical activity and lost less weight. Some women also feel good about exercising because rather than view it is as work, they see it as a social activity—Tuesday is yoga with the girls, for example. Based on 2006 Weight Watchers research, women are far more likely than men to work out with a group of friends or take aerobics classes.

FROM A MAN'S VIEWPOINT
EXERCISE BENEFITS: WEIGHT LOSS AND BEYOND

"No pain, no gain" is a mantra most men have heard somewhere in the course of growing up. While the "no gain" might apply to their weight, most men understand it more in terms of physical results, such as benching more reps or running more miles or showcasing six-pack abs. But it appears that men are starting to tune into the softer benefits of exercise as well. A Stanford University study divided 264 overweight men and women into two groups: those participating in a diet-only weight-loss program and those in a diet-plus-exercise program. The goal was to evaluate the benefits exercise might provide. Compared with men in the diet-only group, men in the diet-plus-exercise program reported feeling less hungry and were better able to follow the diet. The researchers found those results very encouraging, as the newfound benefits are predictive of sustained weight-loss success.

REAL-LIFE LESSON
The Best Exercise Rx

Situation: Ever since I was a young boy, I've always been involved in sports and have exercised. But when I reached my fortieth birthday, I realized I needed to start watching what I ate. I still want to keep exercising, but with a family and a stressful job, it's getting harder to find the time. How much exercise each day is best? I've seen all sorts of numbers—30 minutes, 60 minutes, 90 minutes. Please clarify.

Strategies: Although it may seem that there are a lot of different recommendations for time spent exercising, the confusion lies in believing that being active has only one benefit, and that's not the case. The key is knowing what you expect to achieve with your aerobic exercise regimen and then staying active enough to reach that objective. There are three general benefits that exercise can achieve: health benefits, such as improved mood and blood pressure control; weight loss (in combination with a reduction of food intake); and the prevention of weight gain after a substantial weight loss. The health benefits are obtained with 30 minutes of moderate activity on most (preferably all) days of the week. Weight loss is observed with 45 to 60 minutes. And long-term maintenance of weight loss is associated with levels of 1 hour or more. Knowing what you'll be getting from the time you invest in exercise can help you frame your expectations. And if the hour a day seems impossible right now, don't despair! Finding 30 minutes in your calendar now is the first and most important step. Master that, and you may be surprised by what you'll be able to do in the future. One final recommendation: rather than seeing time with your family as a barrier to exercise, why not turn it into an opportunity? Family activities—from weekend hikes to evening walks to shooting hoops in the back yard—are a terrific way to spend time with the kids, and everyone in the family benefits from the exercise.

Wrapping Things Up

Being physically active is important from both a weight-loss perspective and a health perspective. Women and men, though, approach exercise differently: men give it a higher priority.

- Although it is possible to lose weight by relying solely on exercise, doing so is impractical and unrealistic for most people. Both men and women will achieve greater weight-loss results if they limit the amount of food they eat and exercise regularly.

- To lose weight, men usually turn to exercise first as a way of burning calories, and eventually they discover the importance of limiting their calories from food. Women, on the other hand, typically start by limiting the amount of food they eat and eventually discover the many benefits of exercising.

- Exercise seems to take on a leading role in weight maintenance, preventing lost pounds from returning. Exercise also offers a host of health benefits, including reducing the risk of diabetes, heart disease, premature death, and certain types of cancers. It also improves overall health by strengthening muscles, bones, and joints. And exercise also offers the benefits of stress reduction and an improved mental outlook on life.

Let's Talk!

If you're trying to lose weight with someone of the opposite sex, spend a few minutes evaluating your exercise options. Ask the following questions and see how physical activity can help:

1. What do you think is more important in terms of helping you lose weight: eating less food or exercising?

2. How much time can you spend each day engaged in physical activity? (Make a realistic estimate.)

3. What are some of your favorite physical activities—activities that you can and are willing to do most days of the week?

CHAPTER 10

Support

Everybody Needs Some

John and Kate started dating during their freshman year of college. After graduating, they landed excellent but demanding jobs, John as a CPA at a large accounting firm and Kate as a financial adviser for an investment company. Between their busy careers and active social life, John and Kate find themselves eating out frequently. During the week, they often meet for a quick lunch at a deli near their offices. For dinner they go out or order takeout—pizza or Chinese food. Their weekends are usually jam-packed with social events—attending parties or meeting friends at a sports bar—and that of course leads to more eating out. As a result of their hectic singles lifestyle, good eating and exercise habits have been virtually nonexistent, and each has put on several extra pounds.

After Kate received a huge promotion that required her to spend more time traveling and meeting clients, she decided it was time to update her wardrobe. While she was shopping for new clothes, much to her horror, she discovered that she needed to look for items that were two sizes larger than she expected. Kate vowed that she would not buy anything until she lost some weight.

Kate spent a great deal of time talking with friends and doing research online to figure out what she should do to lose weight. One Web site she found enabled her to calculate her BMI, and she figured out John's as well. The results confirmed what she suspected: with her BMI at 26 and John's at 29, they were both overweight. After talking with a friend who had lost over 50 pounds, Kate decided to join her friend's weight-loss program.

Kate was thrilled with her initial success—she lost 4 pounds in the first 2 weeks. The program taught her several strategies that seemed to help her cut back on her eating. She no longer kept ice cream or desserts in her house; for lunch she started ordering soup and a salad with light dressing on the side; for dinner she ordered steamed Chinese vegetables and she cut down on her alcohol consumption at social events. The approach seemed to work, and the needle on the scale kept heading downward. All her coworkers and friends noticed Kate's progress and were very supportive. They kept telling her how great she looked and asking her to share her secrets.

After losing about 15 pounds, Kate was feeling great—except that she felt John was sabotaging her weight-loss efforts. When they ate out, he ordered dessert. When it was his turn to pick up dinner on the way home from the office, he would arrive at her house with a pizza loaded with pepperoni, sausage, and extra cheese instead of the peppers and onions she had requested. The worst part was that John never commented on how much weight she had lost unless she asked him about it.

Kate was getting discouraged and finding it harder to lose weight. She kept reminding John of his BMI and his need to lose weight, too (he was almost obese). Eventually he agreed to give it a try. Trying to be supportive, Kate offered advice. But her comments ("That's way too big a portion" or "You already had your snack") annoyed him. Any-time she brought up his eating habits or tried to give him guidance on the right way to lose weight, he grew quiet and distant.

One night when they were eating out, John ordered a chocolate-raspberry torte for dessert—Kate's favorite. While they were waiting for the waiter to bring the cake to their table, Kate said, "I thought you said you were going to lose weight! That chocolate cake is loaded with fat and sugar; it's the last thing you need. And since when do you order dessert? You never used to, so why start now? I feel like you're just try-ing to tempt me so that I will gain weight!"

Confused and hurt by Kate's comments, John looked at her and said, "How can you say that? I am happy that you've lost weight and you look terrific! At first I really didn't want to lose weight, but you told me I needed to, so I agreed. I do want to lose weight, but I'm not sure what to do. I know that what you're doing seems to work for you, but it doesn't feel like the right approach for me. I'm too hungry all the time, and you keep telling me what I shouldn't or can't eat. Can you help me figure out what I *can* eat?

Research has identified support as a strong predictor of lasting weight loss for both men and women, but the genders are very different in the types of support they want and the way they go about getting it. Like Kate, many women desire unsolicited verbal support, particularly from their partner—comments about how they look and how well they are doing with their weight loss. While men want verbal support, many guys, like John, are turned off when their mate offers unsolicited feed-back. The majority of guys prefer to be the one who initiates the request for weight-loss help and support.

This chapter explores the gender differences involved in the concept of support and shows how successful couples can be at losing weight if they learn to provide the type of support their partner needs—and avoid giving the type of support they don't like to receive.

Weight Loss: Support Is Key

Fast food, convenience markets, takeout food, vending machines—we live in a ready-to-eat world. Whether you're attending a party, business meeting, or sports event, everywhere you turn, food is lurking. We also live in a technology-friendly world. People don't even have to get up from the couch to change channels on the television or shop for groceries. Although overeating and being inactive are not healthy for anyone, for people in weight-loss mode those are recipes for disaster. How do women and men who are trying to lose weight survive in a too-tempting, too-sedentary environment? They need all

---

Research-Backed Factors Predicting Weight-Loss Success

Factors Linked to Reaching a Weight-Loss Goal

Attending a weight-loss program

Losing weight early in the program

Sticking with the program

Receiving social support

Engaging in regular physical activity

Practicing behavior modification techniques

Monitoring oneself

Setting goals

Factors Linked to Sustainable Weight Loss

Engaging in regular physical activity

Monitoring one's weight and food-related behavior

Developing positive coping skills

Keeping in contact with people who helped with the weight loss

Maintaining normal eating patterns

Seeing improvements in health

Data from Institute of Medicine, *Weighing the Options: Criteria for Evaluating Weight-Management Programs* (Washington, DC: National Academies Press, 1995).

kinds of support. Several studies have identified support as a strong predictor of weight-loss success. In a weight-loss report issued by the Institute of Medicine, a quasi-government nonprofit organization, an expert panel was asked to evaluate all the existing weight-loss research. The report included a summary of the key factors with proven links to weight-loss success. Support was definitely on the experts' list.

What exactly is support? As we saw in chapter 4, it generally means different things to men and women. The sexes do agree, though, on one overall concept about support: when trying to lose weight, support means providing or receiving encouragement, advice, information, and assistance in reaching weight-loss goals. For starters, both women and men require personal support from others, such as doctors, family members, spouses, friends, and coworkers. In addition, many people seek group support through a weight loss program like Weight Watchers. Finally, some people are helped by information and resources provided in books, the Internet, and the news media.

When in weight-loss mode, women and men want verbal as well as physical support. Verbal support involves providing encouraging words and statements like "You are really doing great!" or "I'm proud of you" or "Hang in there!" Keep in mind, though, that providing verbal support can be like walking through a minefield because (as we saw in chapter 4) women and men often use different language to express support. So it's important to be aware of gender-specific phrases when trying to offer support to members of the opposite sex. Both women and men need a more active physical kind of support as well—doing constructive things that help one's partner or friend or family member lose weight. For example, keeping the kitchen cabinets free of trigger foods or snacks and cooking healthy meals are often viewed as supportive gestures.

The bottom line about weight-loss support is that everyone needs it. Both men and women require some verbal and/or active physical support in order to lose weight successfully.

FROM A WOMAN'S VIEWPOINT
WEIGHT LOSS: SUPPORT IS KEY

To lose weight, a guy really counts on his female partner for support—and men will be the first to admit it. But the typical man's idea of support is often different from a woman's. Whereas women often see unprompted verbal comments about their weight-loss efforts as highly supportive (for example, they want a guy to notice that they've lost weight), men tend to look for more practical forms of support. A Weight Watchers study found, for example, that men felt supported when their partner agreed to keep fattening foods out of the house and stocked lower-calorie foods instead.

FROM A MAN'S VIEWPOINT
WEIGHT LOSS: SUPPORT IS KEY

A woman tends to need a lot of verbal and active physical support throughout the weight-loss process, especially from the main man in her life. And based on a Weight Watchers survey, we can surmise that simply noticing a woman's slimmer figure and complimenting her weight-loss success without her prompting the comments encourages most women to stick with their weight-loss plan. Women in the survey said they felt their partners were supportive when they encouraged them to buy new clothes.

REAL-LIFE LESSON
Weight-Loss Etiquette

Situation: My wife and I are both trying to lose weight. Every time we go to a friend's house for dinner, my wife brings some food along that's tasty but not fattening. She says that way we can be sure to have something we can eat. But I feel embarrassed. She says that women bring their own food to dinner parties all the time and that it's a common courtesy. I told her that I think it's rude and that we should eat whatever our friends offer us. Who's right?

Strategies: It's true that taking a dish that fits into your weight-loss plan is an often-used strategy for dealing with social situations in which the food offered may not fit with your plan—the strategy must be working for your wife because she keeps doing it despite your objections. I believe that your dilemma can be fixed by reframing the situation. Clearly, your wife finds safety and security in knowing that she is in control of at least part of the meal when you're dining with friends. That's important to her, and you need to respect that (chances are your hostess respects it, too). At the same time, your embarrassment about showing up with extra food or your own food when you've been invited for a meal is understandable. I suggest that you and your wife make this agreement: at the time your hosts extend an invitation, offer to contribute a dish to the meal. If your wife and the hostess agree that you'll bring the appetizer or dessert or a side dish as part of the meal, you will eliminate the message that seems to be saying, "I need to bring something that I can eat." Instead, you and your wife can feel that you are making a contribution to the meal and are helping the hostess out by taking care of one course of the meal. There's a bonus to you as well. While you're enjoying the dish with your friends, you are enhancing your ability to stick with your weight-loss program.

Where Women and Men Go for Support

When people say they have lost weight on their own, it does not mean that they have lost weight without assistance. In general, women are more likely to seek support from friends, the media, and books. Men, on the other hand, look to their spouse as their main source of support. Why do women often rely on such a variety of resources for help with their weight-loss efforts? Part of the reason revolves around the fact that women have a tendency to be bottom-up thinkers, seeking information and feedback from a variety of sources, so they need support for their weight-loss progress from a variety of sources—from a number of people. If the consensus of friends and colleagues is that they're looking thinner, most women will consider that they are receiving supportive feedback and that others think they are doing well, and they will conclude that they should continue.

Another reason for the female approach to seeking motivation and encouragement from several sources, especially other women, may be traced to gender-specific language barriers on the subject of weight loss (see chapter 4). It's also not uncommon for a woman to view her mate as unsupportive. According to Weight Watchers research, one of the main reasons why many women abandon their weight-loss effort is that they feel their spouse or partner is sabotaging them. This is an interesting finding because in the same survey, when men were asked why they abandoned their weight-loss effort, the concept of sabotage was never mentioned. What did women view as sabotage? Examples of men's sabotaging behavior that the women in the study mentioned include not complimenting the woman on her weight-loss achievements, not expressing pride in her weight-loss effort, and insisting on having fattening foods in the house, which was an especially vexing problem for many women because it violates one of their favorite weight-loss strategies.

Men, on the other hand, are more likely to look to a single source, most often their mate, as a primary source of support. Men tend to be more top-down thinkers or big-picture guys. Consequently, they are less inclined to look to others for comment on their progress. They're more concerned with what the experts think, and men often consider their partner to be an expert. In a study of this topic, men said that they relied on their partners as a source of information about their bodies and that they were more likely to lose weight if their partner thought they needed to. When Weight Watchers asked men in the

United Kingdom about losing weight, the men stated that encouragement from and the involvement of their spouse or female partner was critical to their weight-loss success.

What are the take-away lessons for men and women? For women, seeking weight-loss support from other people and other places is fine, but they want to get support from the men in their lives as well. Where men are concerned, it's great that many of them feel that they need only the women in their lives for weight-loss help, but they need to be aware that there are other resources for motivation and advice out there that can help them achieve success.

FROM A WOMAN'S VIEWPOINT
WHERE WOMEN AND MEN GO FOR SUPPORT

Not all weight-loss programs are created equal. In fact, there are four essential components to look for when selecting a comprehensive weight-loss method. All four components must be in place to ensure successful, lasting weight loss: making wise food choices, being physically active, making positive lifestyle changes, and establishing a supportive environment.

FROM A MAN'S VIEWPOINT
WHERE WOMEN AND MEN GO FOR SUPPORT

Participating in a weight-loss program benefits both women and men. According to a study published in the prestigious *Journal of the American Medical Association*, clear evidence was provided that men and women randomized to follow the Weight Watchers method, with its emphasis on a supportive environment, lost significantly more weight than people assigned to lose weight alone. The two-year study involved over 700 overweight and obese men and women. Over the course of the trial, the participants assigned to attend weekly meetings lost three times more weight than those who dieted on their own. And the more meetings they attended, the more weight they lost!

> **REAL-LIFE LESSON**
>
> **Weight Watchers: Not for Women Only**
>
> *Situation:* My wife has been going to Weight Watchers meetings for the past several months, and she's learned so much about eating smart and losing weight. I'm overweight as well, and she keeps asking me to go with her, but I'm not sure I should join.
>
> *Strategies:* The best way to answer that question is to ask one: What's holding you back? Many men hold the belief that Weight Watchers meetings are a girls-only club and men are unwelcome. Although it is true that more women than men attend Weight Watchers meetings, hundreds of thousands of men attend weekly Weight Watchers meetings all over the world. And don't think that making the decision to join Weight Watchers involves a lot of work and long-term contracts—that's not the case at all. To ease your concerns, why don't you ask your wife about the meetings she attends: Are there men there? Other couples? What goes on in the meeting that might be useful to you? Then try going to a meeting, with or without your wife. You'll be able to see for yourself that the meeting is a lot more about people gathering to learn from one another and the leader and encourage one another's weight-loss efforts than it is about whether you're a man or a woman.

Providing Support: Timing Is Everything

As we discussed earlier in this chapter, scientific evidence confirms something women often have a hard time believing: most men consider them to be weight-loss experts and look to them for help and support. So why do so many women feel that their husbands tune them out when they're offering weight-loss advice? Once again, research provides telling answers. Apparently it's a matter of timing,

Mary Evelyn and Cliff Smith
ONTARIO, CANADA

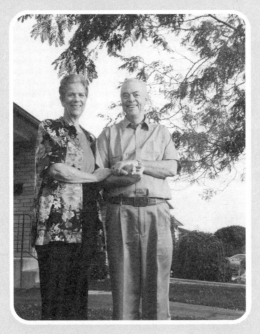

M ary Evelyn and Cliff have been married for about thirty-five years. They have one son, Alfie, who is thirty-three years old. For the past few years, they have been enjoying their retirement, especially now that they have both lost so much weight.

In 1983, Mary Evelyn was in a serious car accident, and one of her ankles was shattered. As a result, she uses a scooter and a wheelchair to get around (although she can stand for short periods of time). According to Mary Evelyn, "Even before my accident, I had been heavy, but after the accident I gained even more weight." She had tried all kinds of diets; once she even lost 100 pounds. But, she says, "That diet was so restrictive that

173

once I had a taste of the forbidden foods, I would go completely out of control and eat nonstop. That type of eating pattern led to wild mood swings and depression until I completely gave up on losing weight. I gained back the 100 pounds I'd lost and put on an additional 100 pounds."

Because of her large size, Mary Evelyn experienced all sorts of problems that prevented her from going out often and socializing with others. She explains, "When I went to restaurants, I couldn't fit into a booth or in an armchair; sitting in a seat in a movie theater was torture; sitting in a lawn chair was scary, especially at other people's houses; and rides at amusement parks were unsafe if the protective bar didn't fit over my stomach. I had to have a special attachment just to buckle my seat belt." Mary Evelyn's health also suffered as a result of her weight. She had high blood pressure and high cholesterol, and she had to take many medicines. She had an excruciatingly painful hernia, but doctors refused to operate because her weight put her at such great risk.

Mary Evelyn felt as if she were at the end of her rope. Then, on October 11, 2002, everything changed. She says, "I was in tremendous pain. Cliff came into the bedroom and told me that we had to do something about my weight because he didn't want to lose me. He was willing to try anything to help me lose weight. We prayed, and then I agreed it was time. I told him that I would get serious and that we needed the best solution, and that I had heard that Weight Watchers was the best. Cliff got out the phone book and called the eight hundred number, and the rest is history."

During the first week, Mary Evelyn lost 6 pounds. Her success motivated her to keep losing. It also motivated Cliff. He says, "I weighed about two hundred fifty-nine pounds, so I was overweight, too. For the most part, I was healthy, but I felt out of breath when I did simple things like when I walked or did yard work." Cliff followed a very restrictive plan, eliminating many kinds of foods from his diet, but he felt hungry all the time. He lost about 50 pounds, but eventually hit a weight-loss plateau.

He says, "After taking Mary Evelyn to her Weight Watchers meetings, I became somewhat envious of her weekly weight-loss success. I was also jealous of all the wonderful foods, fruits, and desserts she got to eat. So I decided to join Weight Watchers, too."

Cliff and Mary Evelyn both follow the Flex Plan. Mary Evelyn says, "I have always been a bridge player, so counting **POINTS**® values was second nature to me." They also started exercising. Cliff loves to walk; Mary Evelyn enjoys swimming. "Being in the water helps me forget that I'm handicapped," she says. And to help his wife with her strength training, Cliff bought equipment and set up a home gym for Mary Evelyn.

Both Cliff and Mary Evelyn are now at their goal weights. Mary Evelyn has lost about 240 pounds and firmly believes that she would never have lost the weight on her own; she relied on Cliff and Weight Watchers for constant support. "The Weight Watchers leaders are so knowledgeable and willing to help," she says, "and Cliff has been my rock; he is so supportive. He never brings junk food into the house to tempt me. In fact, he bought a second refrigerator just to store all our fresh produce."

Cliff says, "When my wife recommended that I join Weight Watchers, I never questioned her judgment. Weight Watchers has taught us both how to eat better." Cliff is also thankful that Mary Evelyn is healthy: she no longer takes any medication and she was able to have the hernia operation. According to Cliff, "We go to the Weight Watchers meetings together. When we are out of town, we look up Weight Watchers meetings that we might be able to attend. And Mary Evelyn uses the message boards on WeightWatchers.com for encouragement and ideas about what to eat." One more thing on which Mary Evelyn and Cliff agree: other than marrying each other, joining Weight Watchers was the best decision they ever made.

and on that score the genders have some fundamental differences. Most men want expert advice, but only when they *ask* for it, whereas most women want unsolicited encouragement, suggestions, and direction from others, including their partner, in support of their weight-loss efforts.

As we saw in chapter 7, men tend to be independent problem-solvers, but only up to a point. Although most guys are reluctant to discuss their problems, when they feel they need more information in order to solve a problem, they do not have an issue with turning to an expert. That problem-solving tactic seems to hold true in the areas of weight loss and support for weight-loss efforts. That's because most guys acknowledge that their female partner typically has more nutrition and weight-loss knowledge than they do. And most guys value and appreciate the information and support a woman can provide—but only if they ask for it.

Unfortunately, when a woman offers unsolicited advice, guys often perceive it as nagging or needling rather than helping. For example, if a woman says, "You should order the grilled salmon; it's the lightest entrée on the menu," her guy may not appreciate her comment. He may think to himself, "There she goes again, ordering my meal as if I don't know what to eat." However, if a man says, "What do you think is the lightest entrée on this menu?" chances are he will happily follow her advice because it is a situation in which he has asked for help.

Why do women tend to offer men unsolicited weight-loss advice? Part of the answer may be that women are eager to help. They think that by sharing their weight-loss knowledge, they are being supportive. But most importantly, many women provide support to guys without being asked because that is how they like to receive support—they make the mistake of assuming that their partner wants to receive support in the same form they want to receive it. While men prefer to ask for help rather than be given an answer to a question they never asked, most women expect others to volunteer feedback, information, and tips that might enable them to lose weight effectively.

For example, if a female coworker says, "I found a Web site that has great recipes that may help you with your weight loss," most women would reply, "Thanks for the tip, I'll check it out." Or if a female neighbor says, "You look fantastic. Have you lost weight?" most women would appreciate that the neighbor noticed the weight loss and would take the remark as a supportive comment.

If women and men really want to support each other's weight-loss efforts, the best strategy is for them to offer the type of support that their partner prefers and at the right time. For women, the best way to show support is to wait until their man asks for it. Men, on the other hand, can show their support by offering sincere compliments and noticing their partner's progress every step of the way.

REAL-LIFE LESSON
Being a Supportive Wife

Situation: Over the past year and half, I have lost about 75 pounds. My husband asked me if I would help him lose weight, too. At first I was more than happy to help him because he needs to lose at least 50 pounds. Every chance I get, I try to tell him what he can and can't eat. And I am always trying to give him advice, even when he doesn't ask for it. Lately, he seems discouraged and not interested in losing weight. Am I doing something wrong?

Strategies: It is obvious that your husband sees you as his weight-loss expert and has asked you to help him lose those 50 pounds. It's terrific that he is aware of his need to shed the excess weight, that he is taking appropriate action to do it, and that he is expanding his resources to include you. You should feel great that he recognizes your success and has sought your counsel. A single request for advice, however, is not an open invitation. If you ask a personal trainer to explain the correct way to do a crunch, you appreciate what he or she has to say, but you might get annoyed if she then gives you information about how to measure your heart rate, stretch your hamstrings, and adjust the seat on your stationary bike (this is an exaggeration to make the point). It seems sensible for you to talk to your husband about what type and how much advice he'd like you to provide. He may want you to help him make a selection from a menu when you're eating out or suggest ideas for lunches when he's at the office. In general, advice is sought to get specific information about a specific issue. As your husband's weight-loss resource, you need to be clear about the problem or problems he's having and limit your advice to those areas—at least until he asks for more advice.

Wrapping Things Up

When it comes to weight loss, the research is very clear: everybody needs support. Support can come from various people, including one's spouse, friends, coworkers, and health professionals. Information can also come from other sources such as books, the Internet, and the news media. Support can also be provided through group support in a weight loss program like Weight Watchers. But the two sexes do have very different points of view when it comes to offering weight-loss support.

- Both women and men need support when they are trying to lose weight. They need verbal support in the form of encouraging comments like "You are doing a great job!" And since actions often speak louder than words, they also need active physical support, such as keeping potato chips out of the house or buying lower-calorie foods.

- Men and women often turn to different people and places for weight-loss support. Women typically rely on friends, coworkers, the media, books, and weight-loss programs. Men, on the other hand, turn to those they perceive as the nutrition and weight-loss expert, and that means most guys turn to their partner as their main source of support.

- One of the fundamental differences between men and women when it comes to providing weight-loss support has to do with timing. Men seek support, particularly from their wives, by asking for it. Women, on the other hand, are very comfortable receiving unsolicited support. Therefore, they often expect their partners to be more forthcoming with verbal and active physical weight-loss support.

Let's Talk!

If you and your partner are both trying to shed extra pounds but have run into some support issues, take a few moments to answer the following questions. Your answers may be the secret to lasting weight loss.

1. Whom do you turn to for weight-loss support and why?

2. What does your partner say or do that you feel hinders (or helps) your weight-loss success?

3. What specific things could your partner say or do to support your weight-loss efforts?

CHAPTER 11

Couples Win the Weight-Loss Race

Family vacation at last! Dave, Cathy, and their two preteen daughters, Chrissy and Lauren, packed up the car; they were looking forward to an action-packed week of roller coasters, water parks, and seven full days of family fun in the sun. They planned to visit several theme parks and wrap up the vacation by spending a few days visiting old friends. Everyone was excited. Cathy had spent days shopping and getting ready for the trip. Since they would be in the car quite a bit, she packed a goodies basket with chips, cookies, candy bars, juice boxes, and sodas to have while they were on the road.

Their first stop was a water park. Chrissy and Lauren could hardly wait to put on their bathing suits and try out the giant slide. While the girls swam, Dave and Cathy sat in the shade enjoying concession-stand cuisine—foot-long hot dogs, cheese fries, and giant-size soft drinks. The girls eventually spotted their parents eating and ran over to ask for food too. Chrissy wanted pizza and Lauren wanted fried chicken fingers.

After eating their fast food feast, the girls headed back to the pool. Dave watched the girls walk away and noticed that they both had rolls of fat that extended beyond the sides of their two-piece bathing suits. He mentioned to Cathy that he thought the girls looked heavier than was healthy. Cathy agreed. She said she'd had a hard time buying clothes for them this year. In fact, she'd had to purchase shorts and dresses in sizes that were too long for the girls and needed to be hemmed. But that was the only option because the clothes that fit lengthwise were too tight around the waist and hips. Dave and Cathy wondered whether they were doing something wrong in the way they were raising their girls and, if so, whether there was something they could do to reverse the situation. Looking back, they realized that their childhoods had been different from those of their daughters. As kids, Dave and Cathy had always been thin, but during her first year of college, Cathy had picked up the infamous freshman 15 pounds. To Cathy's credit, she lost some of the extra college weight after graduation. Then she and Dave got married and they both put on several extra pounds. They continued to gain weight after the girls were born and they settled into a middle-aged family lifestyle. With the demands of work, the kids' schedules, and the busyness of their everyday lives, returning to a healthy weight wasn't a priority for either Dave or Cathy.

After polishing off her last cheese fry, Cathy turned to Dave. She said, "Dave, I have to tell you that I am concerned about all of us! The girls are so much heavier than I was at their age. If I wasn't overweight at their age and I am now, what does that spell for their future? I don't want them to go from being overweight teens to being obese women. And I'm concerned about you, too. I've heard you say that you want to lose weight. Why don't we do it together? Someone told me that when couples work at it together, they're better able to lose weight, and that would be good for the whole family. What do you think?"

Dave thought about it for a few moments, tossed his soda into the trash, and said, "I think you may be on to something. The girls are picking up our eating habits, and obviously they're not very good habits. I want to be a good role model for them. And I know that losing some weight would do me a world of good. I like the idea of our doing it together—we make a great team. And maybe if we start eating healthier and getting more active, the girls will, too."

Dave and Cathy picked up on a proven strategy for weight-loss success: losing weight as a couple. Several studies have confirmed that there are links between a shared home environment and weight. Women and men who live together tend to gain weight at similar times—for example, after getting married and after having children. They also tend to lose weight at similar times. Plenty of research has also found that when women and men tackle weight loss as a couple, they are likely to achieve better results than when they tackle it separately. And since excess weight runs in families, the kids are likely to benefit when their parents have a healthy weight loss because the parents pass on to their offspring their healthier habits of eating better and engaging in physical activity.

Weight is an issue that affects men and women alike. Carrying around extra pounds has an impact on everyone's physical and emotional health, and achieving a healthy weight benefits both sexes. But as we've mentioned, women and men often have different viewpoints about weight and the best ways to take it off. There are valuable lessons to be learned all around; women and men can learn a lot from each other when it comes to lasting weight loss. By understanding and leveraging the differences that exist between the genders, couples can improve their chances of achieving weight-loss success.

Gaining and Losing Weight at the Same Time

While it's true that genetics plays a role in determining body weight, so does living together. Although spouses do not share a gene pool, they do share an environment. And there's a considerable amount of research showing that people who live together, particularly spouses, tend to have similar BMIs. And if that shared environment is encouraging weight gain, there may be an increased risk of obesity. In a study of the relationship between marriage and the development of obesity, researchers followed newly married spouses for two years. At the end of the study, they found that the couples had similar BMIs and that marriage was associated with weight gain. It also appeared that the couples' lifestyle involved eating calorie-laden foods and not engaging in physical activity—and that their newly acquired living arrangement was at least partially to blame for the weight gain.

Why does living together predispose partners to weight gain? The answers fall into two categories. First, marriage generally increases eating opportunities because married people tend to eat together, reinforcing a habit of eating more often. For example, a single woman living on her own may opt for a simple salad for dinner after a busy day at work. Once married and preparing a dinner that she and her husband will share, the woman is more likely to prepare and eat a more complete—and higher-calorie—meal. In addition to having more opportunities to eat with someone, the newly married person may have less motivation to stay thin. In a single world, both men and women want to maximize their attractiveness to the opposite sex, and for many that includes having a trim figure. With marriage, the comfort of being in a stable relationship can lead to a reduced commitment to maintaining one's weight.

Couples are also vulnerable to weight gain after starting a family. This is especially true for women. Several studies have found that childbirth is the primary time of weight gain by women. However, men are also vulnerable to weight gain at this time of life. In one study conducted for Weight Watchers, men between the ages of eighteen and forty-four reported that the birth of their children was a period for significant weight gain.

The evidence is clear: couples who live together tend to gain weight together. That does not mean, however, that the answer to being slim is to avoid marriage! Just as there is research showing that couples tend to gain weight together, there is also evidence that people who share a home are more likely to lose weight at the same time, too. Living in a shared environment in which couples are conscientious about achieving and maintaining a healthy weight often results in a commitment to keeping the kitchen stocked with wholesome, nutritious foods such as fruits, vegetables, lean proteins, low- and nonfat dairy products, and whole-grain breads and pastas. Likewise, the weight-conscious couple is more likely to participate in regular physical activity, either as a couple or singly. This supportive environment is important for both partners, as it creates an atmosphere in which weight loss is encouraged, enabled, and achievable with a minimum of effort.

FROM A WOMAN'S VIEWPOINT
GAINING AND LOSING WEIGHT AT THE SAME TIME

Women are more likely than men to notice an early warning signal when it comes to weight gain, but women also tend to be quicker at taking steps to get rid of a few extra pounds than their male counterparts. If a woman is ready to lose weight and has a partner who would benefit from shedding some pounds, too, is there anything she can do to hasten her mate's weight-loss commitment so that the benefits of doing it together can be realized? Yes, there is, and it doesn't involve talking. In fact, don't say a word—actions speak much louder. Simply follow some of the strategies outlined in chapter 6 to enhance your guy's awareness that he needs to lose weight. For example, send him out shopping for his own clothes so that he can see that he's gone up a size or two—or three. Or make an appointment for him to see his doctor for a physical so that he can hear from an expert how his weight is making him older than his years. The key is getting guys to see that they need to lose weight. When they've made the decision to do it, they will most likely bring up the subject. And since most men consider their partners to be weight-loss experts, chances are they'll come to you for advice and be excited about working with you to create a healthy-weight home.

FROM A MAN'S VIEWPOINT
GAINING AND LOSING WEIGHT AT THE SAME TIME

The downfall for many women is having unrealistic expectations about weight—how much they should weigh and how quickly they'll be able to take the pounds off. That liability can be aggravated when couples are losing weight together. As explained in chapter 5, men have a biological advantage over women when it comes to losing weight—their taller frames and lower body fat help them lose weight more quickly than most women while consuming more calories. To many women, this male advantage can be discouraging.

So how can a guy help the special woman in his life deal with the reality of this gender difference and stay motivated to lose weight? For starters, men need to be sensitive to the biological reality and not say or imply that they are better dieters than their partner. A little empathy can go a long way in evening the playing field in the weight-loss game. To go even further, taking the time to praise a partner's progress with hefty doses of unsolicited support is always appreciated. Comments like "You look fantastic!" or "Why don't you buy a new dress for the holiday party to show off your new figure?" can go a long way toward building the typical woman's commitment to weight loss. Remember: most women need to feel encouraged and supported by their partner in order to maximize their weight-loss success.

REAL-LIFE LESSON

Situation: I have always heard that one's weight is more a matter of genetics than environment. My husband and I are both overweight, and we don't have the most weight-friendly lifestyles. We have an adopted ten-year-old daughter who is thin. Am I right in believing that she is programmed to be a thin adult, so I don't need to pay a lot of attention to what she eats and whether or not she's physically active? I'm assuming that since she's adopted, she's always going to be naturally thin and can't become overweight like my husband and me. Is that right?

Strategies: While it's true that genetics does play a role in weight, it's critical to remember that biology is not destiny. Lots of lean kids grow up to become overweight adults. In fact, most of today's overweight adults were not overweight as children. Most experts agree that genetics can increase the vulnerability to excess weight, but environment is the trump card. The best gift that you can give your daughter, your husband, and yourself is a healthy-weight home environment. As parents, you can be powerful role models for your daughter by taking action and achieving a healthy body weight. By raising her in an environment that supports a lifestyle that includes wholesome, nutritious foods and lots of physical activity, you will be setting the stage for her to grow into a healthy active adult, regardless of whether she has the genes that make it easier or harder to achieve.

Losing Weight as a Couple: Why It Works

When couples join forces to lose weight, the research is very clear—it works! Not only do the partners drop pounds from the bathroom scale, but they often adopt healthier lifestyles and improve their overall health as well.

An innovative study done in Australia demonstrates this reality. The concept was based on the knowledge that the early years of a relationship establish the health- and weight-related habits for decades to come. The researchers designed a study dedicated to affecting positively the lifestyles of couples who were just moving in together—one of the times when couples are most vulnerable to gaining weight. Initially thirty-nine couples participated in a sixteen-week lifestyle-modification program targeted at reversing the weight-gaining trend in new households. As couples, the men and women were taught how to decrease their fat intake and their reliance on fast food and how to increase their physical activity and eat more fruits and vegetables. The results were extremely positive and demonstrated that couples who changed their behaviors as a team had better success than those going it alone. The couples lost weight, ate fewer high-fat foods, and consumed more fruits, vegetables, and reduced-fat foods. They also exercised more and reduced their cholesterol levels by an average of 6 percent.

This first study was so successful that it was expanded to 137 couples. As in the first study, the couples in the follow-up study lost more weight than the control group, experienced similar health benefits, and showed positive lifestyle behavior changes. Most importantly, the results were sustained. One year after the program ended, the couples had maintained their weight loss and improved their health status.

Why is it that couples who choose to lose weight together tend to do better? The answer seems to be the presence of close, constant, and mutual support. Couples help each other get through the challenges that come with losing weight, and they encourage and recognize each other's progress. Whenever lifestyle modification is involved, doing it together makes the most sense.

Take exercise as an example. One study involved married people who were participating in an exercise program. In one group, the married couples did the program together. In the other group was individuals who were married but not participating with their spouse. The results favored the couples. Monthly exercise attendance was significantly higher for the married couples than for the singles: 54 percent compared with 40 percent. And the program dropout rate was dramatically lower as well. Only 6 percent of the married couples dropped out compared with 43 percent of the singles. Half of all the dropouts left because of family responsibilities and lack of spousal support.

Similar results have been found in studies focused on reducing the risk of disease. In a study that involved almost 1,500 British couples who participated in a lifestyle intervention study aimed at reducing the risk factors for cardiovascular disease, researchers were interested in understanding the characteristics of those couples who benefited the most from the program. As part of the program, the couples were encouraged to make changes that would reduce cigarette smoking and lower blood pressure, cholesterol, and blood sugar levels. One year after completing the course, the researchers discovered some interesting results. The people in the study who benefited the most from the program had partners who had also benefited the most. In contrast, the men and women who showed little benefit from the program had partners who also showed little benefit. The researchers concluded that lifestyle programs that targeted men and women as couples rather than as individuals may result in greater cardiovascular improvements.

What does this mean? If you want to improve the odds of weight-loss success and better health, it's worth making the effort to take a team approach.

FROM A WOMAN'S VIEWPOINT
LOSING WEIGHT AS A COUPLE: WHY IT WORKS

As with any team, it's important for the players to know their roles. Here are some of the responsibilities that women may want to lay claim to. First, use the right words. As we saw in chapter 4, language is important, so women need to make sure to use male-friendly words and phrases when they're talking weight loss with their male teammate. Examples include "You look fit" or "What's your weight-loss goal for this week?" Second, do some research. Since women are often viewed by their male partners as the weight-loss expert, it is helpful to gather information that may be useful to the effort. When it comes to learning the details, most guys prefer to punt this responsibility to the ladies. And third, select a weight-loss program that emphasizes cutting calories from food; as chapter 8 points out, that's the major way for anyone to achieve his or her weight-loss goals.

FROM A MAN'S VIEWPOINT
LOSING WEIGHT AS A COUPLE: WHY IT WORKS

When approaching weight loss as a team, each player has to bring his or her best game to the table. Here are some responsibilities that guys can take on to ensure weight-loss victory. Start by being a good communicator. As chapter 4 emphasizes, women and men speak a different weight-loss language. Make sure to provide lots of unsolicited verbal support, using the kinds of words your partner will appreciate most. Comments that will help keep a woman's motivation high include "You look thinner" and "Why don't I make dinner tonight so you'll have time to take a walk?" And when you need some information or advice about a specific challenge you're having, ask the lady in your life to offer her expertise—she's a great resource. Finally, remember that lasting weight loss requires a combination of diet and exercise. Exercise alone is not going to result in a sizeable weight loss, though it's critical for keeping the lost weight off. Make sure that you select an eating strategy that is simple and easy to follow and involves cutting calories.

REAL-LIFE LESSON

Situation: My fiancé and I are getting married in a month. We have heard that many couples gain weight during the first few years of marriage. We don't want that to happen to us. Any suggestions for preventing it from happening?

Strategies: Congratulations on taking a preventive approach to avoiding the honeymoon pounds that so many newly married couples gain. The best advice is to consciously create a weight-friendly environment. This means establishing habits that support weight management, such as eating a wholesome breakfast, establishing and sticking to a regular schedule for physical activity, and planning meals and snacks—and stocking the kitchen with foods—that support a healthy weight. Other suggestions include planning active date nights—for example, go out dancing instead of having dinner at a fancy restaurant—and making a point of regularly complimenting each other on your shared commitment to keeping your newly married physiques!

Weight Loss: A Family Affair

Losing weight as a couple—it's good for each of you, and if you're parents, it can be very good for the kids, too. Two-thirds of adult North Americans are overweight or obese, and the weight statistics for American children are not far behind. Over 9 million children over the age of six are the adult equivalent of obese. And according to the most recent health and nutrition survey, the past thirty years have witnessed a dramatic upward trend in children's weight. The number of overweight children between the ages of two and five has more than doubled; for children between the ages of six and nineteen the number has tripled. Researchers estimate that about 30 percent of children weigh more than they should. Those facts are particularly alarming because research has clearly shown that the likelihood of an overweight child becoming an obese adult is very high. About 33 percent of preschool-age children with excess weight and about 50 percent of

Matt and Martha Suronen
WASHINGTON

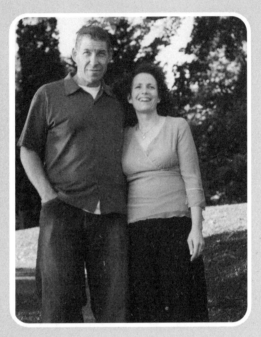

High school sweethearts Matt and Martha have been married for nineteen years. They have two children, Aubery, who is eleven, and Tyler, who is five. Matt works for a health insurance company and Martha is a childbirth educator at the community hospital. Over the years they have watched each other's weight go up and down as if on a roller coaster. In 2003, they made a weight-loss commitment and joined Weight Watchers. Together they have lost over 220 pounds, and they are healthier and more active than they ever were before, even when they were in high school.

Neither Matt nor Martha had a weight problem until college. Matt says, "I didn't gain the freshman fifteen, I gained the freshman forty!" Martha agrees and adds, "And I gained the freshman twenty-five! Even though we would periodically lose some weight, for the most part our weight kept going up. I gained sixty pounds with my first pregnancy. I didn't lose it, and I gained even more with my second pregnancy." Matt was piling on the pounds right along with Martha. He says, "I knew I had gotten big, but I refused to step on a scale because I didn't want to know how much weight I had gained." Unfortunately Matt started experiencing chronic back pain, which his doctors said was weight-related. Matt says, "Martha and I both felt as though we never had any energy to do even simple things like play with the kids or walk up and down steps." Worried about their health (they were only in their mid-thirties) and the negative effect they might have been having on their children, the couple agreed to lose weight, for good this time.

A coworker of Matt's told him about Weight Watchers. Matt joined in January 2003; Martha joined two months later. Martha explains, "I didn't join at the same time Matt did because I had broken my leg in January, and it took a while for me to become mobile enough to leave the house and attend meetings."

According to Matt, joining Weight Watchers was the best weight-loss move he ever made. "I lost twenty pounds right away and became very motivated," he says. One of the things Matt felt helped him lose weight was the initial 10 percent weight-loss goal that Weight Watchers emphasizes. He says, "It was realistic and encouraging because I knew I couldn't lose two hundred pounds, but I could lose twenty." Matt found that setting several mini-goals along the way was very helpful. "I also gave myself rewards for each goal—like five pounds and I could go to the movies," he says. Exercise also became very important to Matt. He started biking and running about 6 months after joining Weight Watchers.

Martha's Weight Watchers experience was also very positive. She says, "I didn't lose weight as quickly as Matt did, but the weight seemed to come off each week a little at a time." The couple started out following the Flex Plan but then switched to the Core Plan. "We have a tendency to go back and forth between the two plans. I like the structure of the Flex Plan, but Matt prefers the Core Plan because he feels that it focuses on wholesome eating, and he can eat as much as he needs to in order to feel satisfied."

Weight Watchers is a lifestyle for their whole family. Martha explains, "We homeschool our kids. Weight Watchers has helped us learn how to be good role models and how to teach our children firsthand about the importance of healthy eating and exercise." So far their approach seems to be working. Both kids are at a healthy weight, and Matt and Martha have each achieved their weight-loss goals. Currently both Matt and Martha are Weight Watchers lifetime members.

school-age children with excess weight become obese adults. In general, children with a high BMI are twice as likely as kids whose BMI is in the healthy-weight range to become obese adults. And the odds shoot up the longer a child's or teen's BMI stays in the at-risk or overweight range.

Despite all the alarming statistics, there is some very good news: parents can help their kids beat the overweight odds by using a healthy approach to weight management themselves. Research has shown that parents who are good nutrition and physical activity role models are more likely to raise kids who are active and have a healthy weight. When it comes to their children's weight, research has found that parents' attitudes and lifestyle practices have a profound effect on their children—and that that effect can be either negative or positive. Even though there is a genetic component to a person's weight, food preferences are largely learned. Indeed, food behaviors have a strong cultural basis and are highly influenced by parents' food choices.

A study that underscores the impact of parental influence on children's food choices analyzed the food preferences of 428 children between the ages of four and five. The families were divided into two groups. In the first group were kids who were at a healthy weight but had overweight or obese parents. In the second group, both the children and their parents were at a healthy weight. For the experiment, parents completed a lifestyle questionnaire and then the children were given a taste test. The researchers found that the children with parents who were overweight or obese had a higher preference for fatty foods in the taste test, a lower liking for vegetables, and a more overeating-type eating style than the kids raised by healthy-weight parents. In addition, the kids in the overweight families had a stronger preference for sedentary activities like watching television, and spent more time engaged in those activities.

Another study highlighting the positive influence parents can have when they are good role models involved increasing families' fruit and vegetable consumption. Researchers found that parents who kept plenty of fruits and vegetables in the home and made it a point to eat them with their children had a positive impact on their children—the kids ate their veggies and fruits, too.

Although it's highly recommended that adults who carry extra pounds lose weight by means of a structured weight-loss plan, experts agree that most children should not be placed on an adult-based weight-loss program. The preferred course of action is for parents to help their children grow into a healthy weight by encouraging them to be more physically active and by improving their overall eating habits. Those goals can best be accomplished when the whole family is involved.

Research has confirmed that family involvement in the weight-loss process has been shown to affect weight-loss success. A study that was designed to improve the eating habits and physical activity levels of Mexican American families showed very promising results for the family-based approach. The researchers divided the families into three groups. The first group was given a booklet about making behavior changes, eating well, and exercising along with a selection of traditional Mexican recipes whose fat content had been modified. The second group was given the same booklet, but in addition a family member was required to attend classes for a year. The third group was given the booklet and the entire family attended classes that emphasized making changes as a family rather than focus on any individual. At the end of the year, the family and the individual groups had significantly greater weight losses than did the booklet-only group, and the family-involvement group had the greatest weight loss.

The take-away message based on years of weight-loss research boils down to this: *Parents, be good role models*. If you have a weight issue yourself, one of the best gifts you can give your children is achieving a healthy body weight by means of a comprehensive lifestyle-based program that helps you to create a healthy-weight home for your entire family. When parents provide their children with a home in which everyone in the family is encouraged to eat well and be active, everyone benefits.

FROM A WOMAN'S VIEWPOINT
WEIGHT LOSS: A FAMILY AFFAIR

Studies have found that mothers tend to feel more responsible than fathers for feeding their children and monitoring their children's diet. But moms who are too concerned about their children's weight and react by limiting the amount of food the child eats may be doing more harm than good. The strategy of restricting or limiting foods often backfires. Kids end up craving and desiring the forbidden foods, and that often leads to overeating—the behavior that Mother was trying to prevent in the first place. Studies have found that providing kids with a variety of foods is the best approach for developing healthy eating habits.

FROM A MAN'S VIEWPOINT
WEIGHT LOSS: A FAMILY AFFAIR

Moms are not the only ones who can influence their children's eating habits; dads can make a big difference, too. Studies are finding that when families—Dad, Mom, and kids—eat meals together on a regular basis, children have fewer problem behaviors. Compared with kids who don't eat regular meals with their families, these kids tend to get better grades in school and are less likely to use drugs. Kids who eat dinner with their families are also at a lower risk of developing an eating disorder. One study found that teens who ate dinner with their family at least three times a week had better eating habits and were less likely to have unhealthy eating behaviors than teens who ate with their family less often. So, dads, make eating dinner together a family priority!

REAL-LIFE LESSON

Situation: Both my wife and I are overweight. We're in the process of trying to lose weight, and so far each of us has lost a few pounds. One reason we're losing weight is so that we can be better role models for our three kids—John, who is ten; Caroline, who is seven; and Peter, who is three. They seem chubby to us. How can we tell if they are overweight? And if they are, what should we do about it?

Strategies: Kudos to you and your wife for taking the right steps toward creating a healthy-weight home for your family. When it comes to kids, it's often difficult to tell whether weight is appropriate simply by looking at them. Even pediatricians have a hard time of it! To get an accurate assessment of how your kids stack up in the weight arena, you need to know their BMI-for-age percentile. You can find this out by asking their pediatrician or consulting the charts provided by the Centers for Disease Control and Prevention at the following Web sites:

For girls: www.cdc.gov/nchs/data/nhanes/growthcharts/
set2clinical/cj41l074.pdf

For boys: www.cdc.gov/nchs/data/nhanes/growthcharts/
set2clinical/cj41l073.pdf

To use the chart, calculate the child's BMI using his or her height and weight (the formula is on the chart). Plotting the BMI for the child's age and gender, the percentile of BMI-for-age shows where the child fits on the weight continuum. A BMI for age above the 85th percentile is equivalent to an adult's being overweight. A BMI-for-age above the 95th percentile is the equivalent of an obese adult.

As for what to do about it, Weight Watchers has published a book that you may find extremely valuable. It's called *Family Power: 5 Simple Rules for a Healthy-Weight Home*, and it's available wherever books are sold.

Wrapping Things Up

Excess weight is an issue that affects both women and men. The good news is that couples can work together to lose the weight and enjoy the many benefits that a healthy weight brings. And doing it together makes good sense.

- When it comes to weight—gaining it and losing it—couples have something in common: they tend to gain and lose weight at the same time. Studies have found that many couples gain weight within their first two years of marriage. One of the key reasons for gaining weight, then, is their shared living environment. But studies have also found that recently married couples who make a concerted effort *not* to gain weight are often successful at keeping the pounds off.

- Women and men who lose weight as a couple are often more successful than women and men who attempt to lose weight on their own. The key to their success seems to be support. Couples who lose weight together tend to help each other more and keep each other's motivation levels high. All of those factors combined seem to increase the odds that they will both meet their weight-loss goals.

- Losing weight as a couple benefits the kids in the family, too. That's because overweight mothers and fathers who lose weight are acting as positive role models for their children. Losing weight as a couple also enables parents to teach their children about the importance of healthy eating and physical activity.

Let's Talk!

Before deciding to lose weight as a couple, ask each other the following questions and use your answers to formulate a weight-loss plan that will work for both of you.

1. When did you notice that you had gained substantial amounts of weight? How do your experiences of gaining weight compare?

2. What are some pros and cons of losing weight together?

3. How are your children affected by your weight, eating habits, and physical activity? In other words, are you a good role model?

CHAPTER 12

Living Healthy

Lifestyle Is Key

On your mark, get set, go! The 10K race began. Judy and Alex took off along with hundreds of fellow runners. This was their third time running in this charity race, an event that was dear to their hearts—the proceeds from the race were being donated to diabetes research. What was most remarkable about Alex and Judy was that five years before, it would have been nearly impossible for either of them to participate in the race. Alex had type 2 diabetes and high blood pressure and was carrying at least 100 extra pounds, particularly in his stomach. Judy had insulin resistance and was at least 75 pounds overweight. Their doctor warned that if they didn't lose weight, their health would continue to decline. He explained that type 2 diabetes is a serious medical condition that can often be prevented or controlled by losing weight and developing healthier eating and exercise habits. That's all Alex and Judy needed to hear. They have two young children who need healthy parents, so they agreed to lose weight together.

Alex and Judy joined a weight-loss program that taught them how to eat a wide variety of nutritious foods and how to incorporate exercise into their lives in a fun and realistic way. After about a year and a half, together they were 175 pounds slimmer. Alex was off all medications, and Judy was given a clean bill of health. For the past several years, they have managed to keep the weight off and have become very active. Every day they have tried to get some type of exercise, whether it is walking, lifting weights, or running. Alex and Judy have enjoyed doing all three of those activities together.

The race was held on a sunny fall morning. Since Alex finished the race a little before Judy, he waited for her at the finish line. While he was waiting, a former neighbor, Bill, came by and said that he had seen Alex's name on the registration list and had been looking all over for him. When Bill couldn't find him, he asked one of the race organizers if he knew where Alex was, and the man had pointed him out. Bill said that he never would have recognized Alex—he looked so fit! Then Bill asked Alex how Judy was doing. Alex spotted her finishing the race and waved for her to join them. Bill commented on how life must be treating them both so well—they were both in such good shape. Bill wanted to know their secret. Alex thought for a moment, then said, "Almost five years ago I had some health trouble and my doctor told me I had to lose weight. Judy was having some health problems, too. We decided that at thirty-eight we were too young to have diabetes, so we joined a weight-loss program and started losing weight together. I've lost about one hundred pounds, and Judy has lost quite a bit too. The best part is that we've been able to keep the weight off for more than three years now. But I'll tell you the truth: I could never have lost this weight on my own. Judy does most of the cooking, and she has taught me so much about what and how much to eat. She is my inspiration and my motivation."

Judy was thrilled to catch up with her old neighbor and to hear Alex compliment her. She said, "Alex is too humble. I had tried to lose weight in the past on my own. I would lose a bit by following one diet or another, but after a while I'd give up the diet and go back to where I was. But not this time. Alex and I have learned how to live a healthier lifestyle. Now that we're in this together, our whole family is healthier—we will never go back to the way we were!"

As we've seen throughout this book, women and men often have very different views about their weight—how they gain it, how they talk about it, and how they think they can lose it. Actually, both genders have strengths and weaknesses in the weight arena. But as chapter 11 highlighted, the research is clear on the benefits of a team approach: losing weight as a couple works. It isn't enough, however, simply to lose weight—keeping it off is at least as important. Having a weight loss that lasts is the ultimate measure of weight-loss success. This chapter reveals the information that can help women and men kiss their extra pounds goodbye for good.

Defining Weight-Loss Success

Men and women have much in common when it comes to defining weight-loss success. Both talk about reaching self-determined weight goals and changing eating behaviors. They differ, however, in rating the importance of keeping the weight off as a defining criterion for success. According to Weight Watchers research, more women than men say that keeping the weight off is very important. Part of the reason may be that men have a tendency to be more successful than women in keeping the weight off. In a national survey conducted for Weight Watchers, significantly more women than men reported regaining weight in the two years after successfully losing weight.

Why is it that in general men seem to be better than women at keeping the lost pounds from reappearing? Some researchers attribute guys' success to their initial motivation to lose weight: health. Men are more likely than women to lose weight in response to a medical event, such as a diagnosis of high blood pressure or high cholesterol (see chapter 6). A study that helps confirm this involved over 900 women and men from the National Weight Control Registry (NWCR). The researchers divided subjects into three groups: those whose weight loss was triggered by medical events, those whose weight loss was triggered by a nonmedical event, and those who reported no triggers. The results revealed that the folks with medical triggers had a greater initial weight loss and gained less weight over two years of follow-up compared to those with nonmedical triggers and no triggers. Also interesting are the overall characteristics of the people in each group. Those with medical triggers tended to be older than those with nonmedical triggers and no triggers (fifty versus forty-four and forty-six years of age, respectively). In addition, in comparison with the other two groups, the participants with medical triggers tended to have the highest BMIs and were more likely to be male compared to those in the other groups. The researchers concluded that medical triggers seem to provide the subjects with lessons about the need to lose weight and may explain why some men have better results than women in terms of initial weight loss and long-term weight maintenance.

FROM A WOMAN'S AND A MAN'S VIEWPOINT
DEFINING WEIGHT-LOSS SUCCESS

The bottom line in defining weight-loss success is that women and men basically use the same definition. Both agree that losing weight and keeping it off are important in defining that success. It's just that since some women seem to experience a little more difficulty than men in keeping the weight off, women often say that they place more importance on weight maintenance. The reality is that weight maintenance is important to both women and men.

> **REAL-LIFE LESSON**
>
> ## Age-Related Weight Gain: Fact or Fiction?
>
> *Situation:* I've always heard that gaining weight as you get older is inevitable. Is that true?
>
> *Strategies:* Although it is true that most people gain weight as they age, it is not inevitable and, most likely, not healthy. The major reason for the weight gain is a change in body composition. As people age, levels of physical activity tend to decline and that, along with some other factors, leads to a gradual reduction in lean body mass. So even at the same weight, a fifty-year-old is likely to have less muscle and more fat than a twenty-five-year-old. Since muscle is the calorie-burning engine of the body, the need for calories to maintain the same weight goes down with age. So if you are fifty years old and you're consuming the same number of calories you consumed when you were twenty-five, you'll gain weight. There is good news, however—by including resistance training in your fitness routine, it is possible to minimize the loss of muscle tissue.

Weight Maintenance: Lifestyle Is Key

When it comes to keeping lost weight off, it's all about maintaining a healthy lifestyle. A large study involving middle-aged men proves this point. The study, which included almost 20,000 men, looked at the impact that some lifestyle changes—such as increasing activity, decreasing time watching television, and improving eating habits—had on weight. Keep in mind that this was not a study that had weight loss as a goal. After four years, the men who adopted the positive lifestyle changes lost an average of about 3 pounds while the men who made no lifestyle changes gained an average of 3 pounds. In addition, the rate of obesity was lowest among those who were physically active compared with those who were sedentary. The researchers concluded that making positive lifestyle changes has the potential to result in modest weight loss or weight maintenance even when weight loss is not a goal.

The National Weight Control Registry, the largest study of individuals successful at long-term maintenance of weight loss, has also provided some outstanding evidence of what it takes to maintain substantial weight loss. The consensus of the NWCR research appears to be that women and men who have been able to lose weight successfully and keep it off have learned to incorporate key positive behavior changes into their lifestyle. Four lifestyle changes common to successful weight losers are consistently making wise food choices, exercising often, regularly eating breakfast, and frequently monitoring one's weight.

Consistently Make Wise Food Choices

A key strategy people use to prevent pounds from reappearing is remaining vigilant about what and how much they eat. The NWCR participants reported consciously choosing foods that are low in calories and low in fat. These folks reported getting an average of 25 percent or less of their daily calories from fat, a strategy that helps to reduce overall caloric intake. Although this level of fat intake is within the recommended range of 20 to 35 percent, it is much lower than what the typical American consumes. However, it's not only the food choices that the NWCR people made that helped them keep the weight off. Making those choices consistently seems to matter, too. These successful weight losers reported maintaining a consistent pattern of eating. In other words, they did not eat differently on weekdays as opposed to weekends, for example.

Exercise Often

As we saw in chapter 9, exercise helps with weight loss, but it appears to be essential to weight maintenance. A whopping 93 percent of NWCR participants reported using some type of physical activity to keep their weight off, with walking being the most popular form of exercise. Twenty-eight percent of participants used only walking as their main form of exercise, while about half used a combination of walking and some other type of planned exercise, such as aerobics classes, swimming, or biking. How much activity did they engage in? NWCR surveys indicate that participants engaged in 60 to 90 minutes of moderate-intensity exercise on most days of the week.

Regularly Eat Breakfast

A large proportion of the NWCR participants reported that they regularly ate breakfast. Seventy-eight percent said that they ate breakfast every day, and only 4 percent said that they never ate breakfast. Based on this information, the researchers concluded that eating breakfast appears to be a positive lifestyle habit, one that seems to play a role in preventing weight gain.

Frequently Monitor One's Weight

NWCR participants said that monitoring their weight by stepping on a scale was something they did frequently. Seventy-five percent of the participants reported weighing themselves at least once a week, and many weighed themselves daily. The researchers concluded that the heightened awareness that came from the participants' staying in touch with their weight seemed to serve as an early warning system for them to take action as soon as they noticed that they had picked up a couple of extra pounds.

If women and men want lasting weight loss, they need to take steps to ensure that the pounds never come back. And according to the research, the best way for both genders to prevent pound rebound is to adopt a healthy lifestyle. The good news is that if weight is lost through a weight-loss approach that is based on lifestyle modification, the changes that are needed to maintain the weight loss have already been learned and engrained into one's everyday life.

According to the NWCR data, about 42 percent of the people who were able to lose weight successfully felt that maintaining their weight loss was less difficult than losing the weight. Why might that be? Studies have found that the longer one practices a healthy lifestyle, the more pleasurable it becomes. Certainly, maintaining a healthy lifestyle is easier when it's the norm in the house and couples are working together toward the same goal. The message seems to be clear: women and men who have lost weight together will want to continue maintaining a healthy lifestyle so that they can maintain their weight loss together.

Wrapping Things Up

Achieving lasting weight loss is not easy, but there are ways to make the process easier. One way is to make lifestyle modification the foundation of any approach used to get the weight off and reach a healthy body weight. What is meant by lifestyle modification? When it comes to weight, it means four things:

- making wise food choices
- being physically active
- developing strong thinking skills, including stress management techniques, coping strategies, and time management expertise, that buttress the ability to eat well and stay active
- creating a supportive environment that includes both personal relationships and physical space

There is no question that healthy living leads to a healthy weight and that modifying one's lifestyle to align with a healthy weight is essential to long-term weight management.

A second way to make the process of weight loss and maintenance easier is to enlist the help of others. While assistance from a variety of

Lydia and Martin Jansen
WISCONSIN

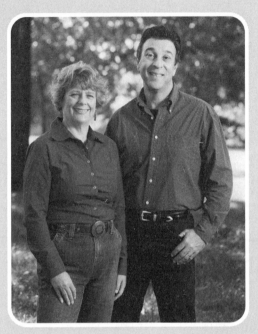

Lydia and Martin, who are in their late forties, have very busy careers and home lives. Martin works as a computer analyst for a local health insurance company; Lydia is a trainer for a financial institution, and her job requires her to travel frequently. They have two teenage children, John and Jill (who is the spitting image of Lydia), and both kids are involved in high school activities. Martin and Lydia also volunteer on weekends to cantor for their church.

In 2003, Martin's doctor was concerned about his low iron levels (he turned out to be anemic), lack of exercise, and weight. Based on his doctor's recommendation, Martin spent the next year trying to exercise. He says, "I lost about twenty pounds, but my weight loss just seemed to stall." Meanwhile, Lydia, who was born with a defective hip, had also put on about thirty extra pounds. She explains, "I'd never had a weight problem before, but the hip was limiting my mobility." In early 2004, Lydia had hip replacement surgery. Her doctor told her that she had to keep her weight down if she wanted to avoid a second hip-replacement operation in the future.

Determined to lose weight and keep it off, Lydia researched her options thoroughly. She says, "My sister and brother-in-law had impressive results on the Weight Watchers program. They each lost forty to fifty pounds." So Lydia decided to join Weight Watchers as well. "I reached my goal weight four months later," she says.

While Lydia was going to Weight Watchers, Martin was looking over her shoulder. He explains, "I noticed her tremendous success, so I decided to join Weight Watchers, too. That way we could go to the meetings together. Weight Watchers helped me lose about twenty-one pounds and reach my goal weight within the first year."

Currently Martin and Lydia are lifetime members. They follow the Flex Plan and still attend weekly meetings together. In addition, they have become avid cyclists and even bike to meetings. Martin says, "Weight Watchers has become a way of life for us, even for our children." Lydia says, "Martin and I work as a team. We consult each other about meals and plan what we're going to eat. If I'm out of town, I try to make sure there are a few healthy meals on hand. One of our family favorites is tacos. I usually keep two fillings handy so the family can just heat and eat." Martin adds, "We are both accountable for the grocery shopping. Weight Watchers has taught me how to be a better label reader. Now it's easy to go to the store and buy healthy and tasty food."

Both Martin and Lydia have kept their weight off for almost two years. They agree that the key to their weight-loss success was doing it together. Martin says, "If Lydia wasn't doing this with me, I would probably have gained back the weight long ago." Martin and Lydia keep tabs on each other to make sure they don't gain the weight back—and as busy as they both are, they find time to attend weekly Weight Watchers meetings and exercise daily. Lydia sums up their commitment perfectly: "Weight Watchers is a natural part of our life now and forever."

people—including coworkers and peers in a weight-loss group—can make a huge difference, there is one person who can make all the difference.

Who's in the best position to assist in the creation of a supportive environment? The person with whom you have the most intimate personal relationship and with whom you live every day. And the ultimate supportive environment is a home in which both partners are committed to achieving and maintaining a healthy weight. Assuming that the partners sharing a home are different genders, there are additional benefits to be gained. The purpose of this book is to break through the weight barriers between the sexes and point the way toward realizing the synergies to be gained by taking a couple's approach to weight loss.

The third way to make the process of weight loss and maintenance easier is to participate in a comprehensive weight-loss program, preferably one that is meeting-based. Weight Watchers research has scientific proof that its method of lifestyle modification that includes weekly meetings results in significantly greater weight loss and weight maintenance than a self-directed approach. It makes sense that those results can be enhanced if a couple committed to losing weight together also participate in the weight-loss program together. Research has shown that people who participate in a weight-loss program and attend weekly meetings with friends and family members are more successful than those who go solo.

Excess weight is an issue that affects men and women—physically and emotionally. By joining forces, couples can tackle their problem pounds as a team, and although it may not be easy, it will definitely be easier doing it together. And it is well worth the effort!

Sources

List of Abbreviations

Am J Clin Nutr	*American Journal of Clinical Nutrition*
Am J Epidemiol	*American Journal of Epidemiology*
Am J Physiol	*American Journal of Physiology*
Am J Public Health	*American Journal of Public Health*
Ann Intern Med	*Annals of Internal Medicine*
Appetite	*Appetite*
Arch Fam Med	*Archives of Family Medicine*
Arch Intern Med	*Archives of Internal Medicine*
Arq Bras Cardiol	*Arquivos Brasileiros de Cardiologia*
Asia Pac J Clin Nutr	*Asia Pacific Journal of Clinical Nutrition*
Basic Appl Soc Psych	*Basic and Applied Social Psychology*
Cancer Epidemiol Biomarkers Prev	*Cancer, Epidemiology, Biomarkers & Prevention*
CMAJ	*Canadian Medical Association Journal*
Cent Eur J Public Health	*Central European Journal of Public Health*
Circulation	*Circulation*
Diabetes Care	*Diabetes Care*

Diabetes Res Clin Pract	*Diabetes Research and Clinical Practice*
Eat Behav	*Eating Behaviors*
Eat Disord	*Eating Disorders*
Eat Weight Disord	*Eating and Weight Disorders*
Epidemiology	*Epidemiology*
Fam Pract	*Family Practice*
Food Review	*Food Review*
Gynecol Obstet Invest	*Gynecologic and Obstetric Investigation*
Health Care Women Int	*Health Care for Women International*
Health Educ Behav	*Health Education & Behavior*
Health Educ Res	*Health Education Research*
Hum Reprod	*Human Reproduction*
Int J Eat Disord	*International Journal of Eating Disorders*
Int J Obes Relat Metab Disord	*International Journal of Obesity and Related Metabolic Disorders*
J Abnorm Psychol	*Journal of Abnormal Psychology*
JAMA	*Journal of the American Medical Association*
J Adolesc Health	*Journal of Adolescent Health*
J Am Diet Assoc	*Journal of the American Dietetic Association*
J Androl	*Journal of Andrology*
J Cardiopulm Rehabil	*Journal of Cardiopulmonary Rehabilitation*
J Consult Clin Psychol	*Journal of Consulting and Clinical Psychology*
J Health Psychol	*Journal of Health Psychology*
J Natl Cancer Inst	*Journal of the National Cancer Institute*
J Nutr	*Journal of Nutrition*
J Nutr Health Aging	*Journal of Nutrition, Health and Aging*
J Per Soc Psychol	*Journal of Personality and Social Psychology*

J Psychosom Res	*Journal of Psychosomatic Research*
Med Sci Sports Exerc	*Medicine and Science in Sports and Exercise*
MMWR	*Centers for Disease Control and Prevention—Morbidity and Mortality Weekly Report*
N Eng J Med	*New England Journal of Medicine*
Obesity	*Obesity*
Obes Res	*Obesity Research*
Pediatrics	*Pediatrics*
Pers Individ Dif	*Personality and Individual Differences*
Physiol Behav	*Physiology and Behavior*
Prev Med	*Preventive Medicine*
Psychiatr Clin North Am	*Psychiatric Clinics of North America*
Psychol Med	*Psychological Medicine*
Public Health Nutr	*Public Health Nutrition*
Reprod Biomed Online	*Reproductive Biomedicine Online*
Sex Roles	*Sex Roles*
Ugeskr Laeger	*Ugeskrift for Laeger*

Chapter 1. Weight Is Not Just a Female Issue

Abernathy RP, Black DR. Healthy body weights: an alternative perspective. *Am J Clin Nutr.* 1996; 63: S448–51.

Blehar MC. Public health context of women's mental health research. *Psychiatr Clin North Am.* 2003; 26: 781–99.

Brady KT, Randall CL. Gender differences in substance use disorders. *Psychiatr Clin North Am.* 1999; 22: 241–52.

Bray GA. *Contemporary Diagnosis and Management of Obesity,* 2nd ed. Newton, PA: Handbooks in Health Care Company, 2003.

Ellis L. Gender differences in smiling: an evolutionary neuroandrogenic theory. *Physiol Behav.* 2006; 88: 303–8.

Gray J. *Men Are from Mars, Women Are from Venus.* New York: HarperCollins, 1992.

McArdle WD, Katch FI, Katch VL. *Sports and Exercise Nutrition*, 2nd ed. Baltimore: Lippincott Williams & Wilkins, 2005.

Ogden CL, Carroll MD, Curtin LR, McDowell MA, Tabak CJ, Flegal KM. Prevalence of overweight and obesity in the United States, 1999–2004. *JAMA.* 2006; 295: 1549–55.

Petersson BH. Gender—an important parameter in medical science. *Ugeskr Laeger.* 1993; 155: 1887–8.

Chapter 2. The Weight-Health Connection: How the Genders Differ

Allison DB, Hoy MK, Fournier A, Heymsfield SB. Can ethnic differences in men's preferances for women's body shapes contribute to ethnic differences in female adiposity? *Obes Res.* 1993; 1: 425–32.

Anderson JW, Konz EC. Obesity and disease management: effects of weight loss on comorbid conditions. *Obes Res.* 2001; 4: S326–34.

Andersson SO, Wolk A, Bergstrom R, Adami HO, Enghold G, Englund A, Nyren O. Body size and prostate cancer: a 20-year follow-up study among 135,006 Swedish construction workers. *J Natl Cancer Inst.* 1997; 89: 385–9.

Bray GA. *Contemporary Diagnosis and Management of Obesity*, 2nd ed. Newton, PA: Handbooks in Health Care Company, 2003.

Brownell KD, Wadden TA. Etiology and treatment of obesity: understanding a serious, prevalent, and refractory disorder. *J Consult Clinl Psychol.* 1992; 60: 505–17.

Cash TF, Prunzinsky T. *Body Images: Development, Deviance, and Change.* New York: Guilford Press, 2004.

Chan JM, Rimm EB, Colditz GA, Stampfer MJ, Willet WC. Obesity, fat distribution, and weight gain as risk factors for clinical diabetes in men. *Diabetes Care.* 1994; 17: 961–9.

Choi HK, Atkinson K, Karlson EW, Curhan G. Obesity, weight change, hypertension, diuretic use, and risk of gout in men: the health professionals follow-up study. *Arch Intern Med.* 2005; 165: 742–8.

Clark AM, Thornley B, Tomlinson L, Galletley C, Norman RJ. Weight loss in obese infertile women results in improvement in reproductive outcome for all forms of fertility treatment. *Hum Reprod.* 1998; 13: 1502–5.

Clinical Guidelines on the Identifcation, Evaluation, and Treatment of Overweight and Obesity in Adults: The Evidence Report. Accesssed online October 7, 2006, at www.nhlbi.nih.gov/guidelines/obesity/

Colditz GA, Willet WC, Rotnitzky A, Manson JE. Weight gain as a risk factor for clinical diabetes mellitus in women. *Ann Intern Med.* 1995; 122: 481–6.

Crandall CS. Prejudice against fat people: ideology and self-interest. *J Per Soc Psychol.* 1994; 66: 882–94.

Dixon JB, Dixon ME, O'Brien PE. Depression in association with severe obesity: changes with weight loss. *Arch Intern Med.* 2003; 163: 2058–65.

Esposito K, Giugliano F, Di Palo C, Giugliano G, Marfella R, D'Andrea F, D'Armiento M, Giugliano D. Effect of lifestyle changes on erectile dysfunction in obese men: a randomized controlled trial. *JAMA.* 2004; 291: 2978–84.

Gardner RM, Martinez R, Sandoval Y. Obesity and body image: an evaluation of sensory and non-sensory components. *Psychol Med.* 1987; 17: 927–32.

Glazer NL, Hendriskson AF, Schellenbaum GD, Mueller BA. Weight change and the risk of gestational diabetes in obese women. *Epidemiology.* 2004; 15: 733–7.

Gluck ME, Geliebter A. Racial/ethnic differences in body image and eating behaviors. *Eat Behav.* 2002; 3: 143–51.

Grogan S. *Body Image.* London: Routledge, 1999.

Harvie M, Howell A, Vierkant RA, Kumar N, Cerhan JR, Kelemen LE, Folsom AR, Sellers TA. Association of gain and loss of weight before and after menopause with risk of postmenopausal breast cancer in the Iowa women's health study. *Cancer Epidemiol Biomarkers Prev.* 2005; 14: 656–61.

Hebl MR. The stigma of obesity: what about men? *Basic Appl Soc Psych.* 2005; 27: 267–75.

Hoffman JM, Brownell KD. Sex differences in the relationship of body fat distribution with psychosocial variables. *Int J Eat Disord.* 1997; 22: 139–45.

Klem ML, Wing RR, McGuire MT, Seagle HM, Hill JO. A descriptive study of individuals successful at long-term maintenance of substantial weight loss. *Am J Clin Nutr.* 1997; 66: 239–46.

Koh-Banerjee P, Wang Y, Hu FB, Spiegelman D, Willett WC, Rimm EB. Changes in body weight and body fat distribution as risk factors for clinical diabetes in US men. *Am J Epidemiol.* 2004; 159: 1150–9.

Kort HI, Massey JB, Elsner CW, Mitchell-Leef D, Shapiro DB, Witt MA, Roudebush WE. Impact of body mass index values on sperm quantity and quality. *J Androl.* 2006; 27: 450–2.

Kumanyika S, Wilson JF, Guilford-Davenport M. Weight related attitudes and behaviors of black women. *J Am Diet Assoc.* 1993; 93: 416–22.

Li Ty, Rana JS, Manson JE, Willet WC, Stampfer MJ, Colditz GA, Rexrode KM, Hu FB. Obesity as compared with physical activity in predicting risk of coronary heart disease in women. *Circulation.* 2006; 113: 499–506.

Lowe MR, Miller-Kovach K, Frye N, Phelan S. An initial evaluation of a commercial weight loss program: short-term effects on weight, eating behavior, and mood. *Obes Res.* 1999; 7: 51–9.

Mahan KL, Escott-Stump S, eds. *Krause's Food and Nutrition, and Diet Therapy,* 11th ed. New York: Saunders, 2003.

Matsuzawa Y, Shimomura I, Nakamura T, Keno Y, Tokunaga K. Pathophysiology and pathogenesis of visceral fat obesity. *Diabetes Res Clin Pract.* 1994; 24: S111–6.

McArdle WD, Katch FI, Katch VL. *Sports and Exercise Nutrition,* 2nd ed. Baltimore: Lippincott Williams & Wilkins, 2005.

Mertens IL, Van Gaal LF. Overweight, obesity, and blood pressure: the effects of modest weight reduction. *Obes Res.* 2000; 8: 270–8.

Min JK, Williams KA, Okwuosa TM, Bell GW, Panutich MS, Ward RP. Prediction of coronary heart disease by erectile dysfunction in men referred for nuclear stress testing. *Arch Intern Med.* 2006; 166: 201–6.

Ogden CL, Carroll MD, Curtin LR, McDowell MA, Tabak CJ, Flegal KM. Prevalence of overweight and obesity in the United States, 1999–2004. *JAMA.* 2006; 295: 1549–55.

Oguma Y, Sesso HD, Paffenbarger RS Jr, Lee IM. Weight change and risk of developing type 2 diabetes. *Obes Res.* 2005; 13: 945–51.

Ostovich JM, Rozin P. Body image across three generations of Americans: inter-family correlations, gender differences, and generation differences. *Eat Weight Disord.* 2004; 9: 186–93.

Pasquali R, Gambineri A. Role of changes in dietary habits in polycystic ovary syndrome. *Reprod Biomed Online.* 2004; 8: 431–9.

Ramirez EM, Rosen JC . A comparison of weight control and weight control plus body image therapy for obese men and women. *J Consult Clin Psychol.* 2001; 69: 440–6.

Rippe JM, Price JM, Hess SA, Kline G, DeMers KA, Damitz S, Kreidieh I, Freedson P. Improved psychological well-being, quality of life, and health practices in moderately overweight women participating in a 12-week structured weight loss program. *Obes Res.* 1998; 6: 208–18.

Rodriguez C, Patel AV, Calle EE, Jacobs EJ, Chao A, Thun MJ. Body mass index, height, and prostate cancer mortality in two large cohorts of adult men in the United States. *Cancer Epidemiol Biomarkers Prev.* 2001; 10: 345–53.

Smith DE, Thompson JK, Raczynski JM, Hilner JE. Body image among men and women in a biracial cohort: the CARDIA Study. *Int J Eat Disord.* 1999; 25: 71–82.

Sorbara M, Geliebter A. Body image disturbance in obese outpatients before and after weight loss in relation to race, gender, binge eating, and age of onset of obesity. *In J Eat Disord.* 2002; 31: 416–23.

Tiggeman M, Rothblum ED. Gender differences in social consequences of perceived overweight in the United States and Australia. *Sex Roles.* 1988; 18: 75–86.

2005 Dietary Guidelines Advisory Committee Report. Accessed online October 3, 2006, at www.healthierus.gov/dietaryguidelines/

van Swieten EC, van der Leeuw-Harmsen L, Badings EA, van der Linden PJ. Obesity and clomiphene challenge test as predictors of outcome of in vitro fertilization and intracytoplasmic sperm injection. *Gynecol Obstet Invest.* 2005; 59: 220–4.

Wannamethee SG, Shaper AG. Weight change and duration of overweight and obesity in the incidence of type 2 diabetes. *Diabetes Care.* 1999; 22: 1266–72.

Weinstein AR, Sesso HD, Lee IM, Cook NR, Manson JE, Burning JE, Gaziano JM. Relationship of physical activity vs body mass index with type 2 diabetes in women. *JAMA.* 2004; 292: 1188–94.

Wing RR, Epstein LH, Marcus MD, Kupfer DJ. Mood changes in behavioral weight loss programs. *J Psychosom Res.* 1984; 28: 189–96.

Zellner DA, Harner DE, Adler RL. Effects of eating abnormalities and gender on perceptions of desirable body shape. *J Abnorm Psychol.* 1989; 98: 93–6.

Chapter 3. When and How the Mirror Lies

Cachelin FM, Striegel-Moore RH, Elder KA. Realistic weight perception and body size assessment in a racially diverse community sample of dieters. *Obes Res.* 1998; 6: 62–8.

Centers for Disease Control and Prevention (CDC). *Behavioral Risk Factor Surveillance System Survey Data.* Atlanta, Georgia: U.S. Department of Health and Human Services, Centers for Disease Control and Prevention, 1996 and 2000.

Green KL, Cameron R, Polivy J, Cooper K, Liu L, Lieter L, Heatherton T. Weight dissatisfaction and weight loss attempts among Canadian adults. Canadian Heart Health Surveys Research Group. *CMAJ.* 1997; 157: S17–25.

Kuchler F, Variyam JN. Mistakes were made: misperception as a barrier to reducing overweight. *Int J Obes Relat Metab Disord.* 2003; 27: 856–61.

Ogden CL, Carroll MD, Curtin LR, McDowell MA, Tabak CJ, Flegal KM. Prevalence of overweight and obesity in the United States, 1999–2004. *JAMA.* 2006; 295: 1549–55.

Paeratakul S, White MA, Williamson DA, Ryan DH, Bray GA. Sex, race/ethnicity, socioeconomic status, and BMI in relation to self-perception of overweight. *Obes Res.* 2002; 10: 345–50.

Rand CSW, Resnick JL. The "good enough" body size as judged by people of varying age and weight. *Obes Res.* 2000; 8: 309–16.

Serdula MK, Mokdad AH, Williamson DF, Galuska DA, Mendlein JM, Health GW. Prevalence of attempting weight loss and strategies for controlling weight. *JAMA.* 1999; 282: 1353–8.

Chapter 4. He's Fit, She's Thin: The Language of Weight Loss

Prochaska JO, Norcross J, DiClemente, C. *Changing for Good.* New York: Avon Books, 1994.

Chapter 5. Why Guys Lose Weight Faster

Behnke AR. *Evaluation and Regulation of Body Build and Composition.* Englewood Cliffs, NJ: Prentice Hall, 1974.

Carpenter WH, Fonong T, Toth MJ, Ades PA, Calles-Escandon J, Walston JD, Poehlman ET. Total daily energy expenditure in free-living older African-Americans and Caucasians. *Am J Physiol.* 1998; 274: E96–101.

Institute of Medicine of the National Academies. *Nutrition During Pregnancy: Part I: Weight Gain, Part II: Nutrient Supplements.* Washington, DC: National Academies Press, 1990.

Janssen I, Ross R. Linking age-related changes in skeletal muscle mass and composition with metabolism and disease. *J Nutr Health Aging.* 2005; 9: 408–19.

Mahan KL, Escott-Stump S, eds. *Krause's Food and Nutrition, and Diet Therapy,* 11th ed. New York: Saunders, 2003.

McArdle WD, Katch FI, Katch VL. *Sports and Exercise Nutrition,* 2nd ed. Baltimore: Lippincott Williams & Wilkins, 2005.

Mirzadehgan P, Harrison GG, DiSogra C. *Nearly One in Five California Adults Obese and Most Still Gaining Weight.* Fact Sheet, UCLA Center for Health Policy Research, December 2004. Accessed online October 7, 2006 at www.healthpolicy.ucla.edu

Ross R, Dagnone D, Jones PJ, Smith H, Paddags A, Hudson R, Janssen I. Reduction of obesity and related comorbid conditions after diet-induced weight loss or exercise-induced weight loss in men. A randomized, controlled trial. *Ann Intern Med.* 2000; 133: 92–103.

Sammel MD, Grisso JA, Freeman EW, Hollander L, Liu L, Liu S, Nelson DB, Battistini M. Weight gain among women in the late reproductive years. *Fam Pract.* 2003; 20: 401–9.

Saris WH. Fit, fat, and fat free: the metabolic aspects of weight control. *Int J Obes Relat Metab Disord.* 1998; 2: S15–21.

Wing RR, Matthews KA, Kuller LH, Meilahn EN, Plantinga PL. Weight gain at the time of menopause. *Arch Intern Med.* 1991; 151: 97–102.

Chapter 6. Dress Sizes, Belt Notches, and Other Weight-Loss Triggers: Why We Lose Weight

Allan JD. To lose, to maintain, to ignore: weight management among women. *Health Care Women Int.* 1991; 12: 223–5.

Carpentar KM, Hasin DS, Allison DB, Faith MS. Relationships between obesity and DSM-IV major depressive disorder, suicide ideation, and suicide attempts: results from a general population study. *Am J Public Health.* 2000; 90: 251–7.

Dallongeville J, Marecaux N, Cottel D, Bingham A, Amouyel P. Association between nutrition knowledge and nutritional intake in middle-aged men from Northern France. *Public Health Nutr.* 2001; 4: 27–33.

De Souza P, Ciclitira KE. Men and dieting: a qualitative analysis. *J Health Psychol.* 2005; 10: 793–804.

Fiala J, Brazdova Z. A comparison between the lifestyles of men and women—parents of school age children. *Cent Eur J Public Health.* 2000; 8: 94–100.

Hawkins N, Richards P, Granley H, Stein D. The impact of exposure to the thin-ideal media image on women. *Eat Disord.* 2004; 12: 35–50.

Parmenter K, Waller J, Wardle J. Demographic variation in nutrition knowledge in England. *Health Educ Res.* 2000; 15: 163–74.

Rippe JM. *Weight Watchers Weight Loss That Lasts.* Hoboken, NJ: John Wiley & Sons, 2005.

Wing RR, Phelan S. Long-term weight loss maintenance. *Am J Clin Nutr.* 2005; 82: S222–5.

Chapter 7. How We Lose Weight:
The Two Sexes Do It Differently

Canadian Statistics Selected Leading Causes of Death, by Sex. Accessed online October 2, 2006, at www.40statcan.ca

CDC National Center for Health Statistics Deaths—Leading Causes. Accessed online October 2, 2006, at www.cdc.gov.

Methods for voluntary weight loss and control. *NIH Technol Assess Conf Statement.* 1992, March 30–Apr 1. Bethesda, MD: National Institutes of Health, Office of Medical Applications of Research.

Ogden CL, Carroll MD, Curtin LR, McDowell MA, Tabak CJ, Flegal KM. Prevalence of overweight and obesity in the United States, 1999–2004. *JAMA.* 2006; 295: 1549–55.

Chapter 8. Women and Men Need to Eat Fewer
Calories: What Works and What Doesn't

Brown MJ, Ferruzzi MG, Nguyen ML, Cooper DA, Eldridge AL, Schwartz SJ, White WS. Carotenoid bioavailability is higher from salads ingested with full-fat than with fat-reduced salad dressings as measured with electrochemical detection. *Am J Clin Nutr.* 2004; 80: 396–403.

Centers for Disease Control. Trends in intake of energy and macronutrients—United States, 1971–2000. *MMWR.* 2004; 53: 80–2.

Chanmugam P, Guthrie JF, Cecilio S, Morton JF, Basiotis PP, Anand R. Did fat intake in the United States really decline between 1989–1991 and 1994–1996? *J Am Diet Assoc.* 2003; 103: 867–72.

DellaValle DM, Roe LS, Rolls BJ. Does the consumption of caloric and non-caloric beverages with a meal affect energy intake? *Appetite.* 2005; 44: 187–93.

Dube L, LeBel J, Lu J. Affect asymmetry and comfort food consumption. *Physiol Behav.* 2005; 86: 559–67.

Himaya A, Louis-Sylvestre J. The effect of soup on satiation. *Appetite.* 1998; 30: 199–210.

Mattes R. Soup and satiety. *Physiol Behav.* 2005; 83: 739–47.

Nielsen SJ, Siega-Riz AM, Popkin BM. Trends in energy intake in U.S. between 1977 and 1996: similar shifts seen across age groups. *Obes Res.* 2002; 10: 370–8.

Putnam J, Allshouse J, Scott Kantor L. U.S. per capita food supply trends: more calories, refined carbohydrates, and fats. *Food Review.* 2002; 25: 2–15.

Smiciklas-Wright H, Mitchell DC, Mickle SJ, Goldman JD, Cook A. Foods commonly eaten in the United States, 1989–1991 and 1994–1996: Are portion sizes changing? *J Am Diet Assoc.* 2003; 103: 41–7.

Rolls BJ, Roe LS, Meengs JS. Salad and satiety: energy density and portion size of a first-course salad affect energy intake at lunch. *J Am Diet Assoc.* 2004; 104: 1570–6.

Rolls BJ, Roe LS, Meengs JS. Larger portion sizes lead to a sustained increase in energy intake over 2 days. *J Am Diet Assoc.* 2006; 106: 543–9.

Rolls BJ, Bell EA, Thorwart ML. Water incorporated into a food but not served with a food decreases energy intake in lean women. *Am J Clin Nutr.* 1999; 70: 448–55.

Young LR, Nestle M. Expanding portion sizes in the U.S. marketplace: implications for nutrition counseling. *J Am Diet Assoc.* 2003; 103: 231–4.

Zizza C, Siega-Riz Am, Popkin BM. Significant increase in young adults' snacking between 1977–1978 and 1994–1996 represents a cause for concern! *Prev Med.* 2001; 32: 303–10.

Chapter 9. Move More to Keep It Off

Centers for Disease Control and Prevention Physical Activity for Everyone: Physical Activity Terms. Accessed online October 2, 2006, at www.cdc.gov/nccdphp/dnpa/physical/terms/

Cox KL, Burke V, Morton AR, Beilin LJ, Puddley IB. Independent and additive effects of energy restriction and exercise on glucose and insulin concentrations in sedentary overweight men. *Am J Clin Nutr.* 2004; 80: 308–16.

Davis C, Elliot S, Dionne M, Mitchell I. The relationship of personality factors and physical activity to body dissatisfaction in men. *Person Individ Dif.* 1991; 12: 689–94.

Gallagher KI, Jakicic JM, Napolitano MA, Marcus BH. Psychosocial factors related to physical activity and weight loss in overweight women. *Med Sci Sports Exerc.* 2006; 38: 971–80.

Jakicic JM. The role of physical activity in prevention and treatment of body weight gain in adults. *J Nutr.* 2002; 132: S3826–9.

Jakicic JM, Clark K, Coleman E, Donnelly JE, Foreyt J, Melanson E, Volek J, Volpe SL, American College of Sports Medicine. American College of Sports Medicine position stand. Appropriate intervention strategies for weight loss and prevention of weight regain for adults. *Med Sci Sports Exerc.* 2001; 33: 214–56.

Jakicic JM, Polley BA, Wing RR. Accuracy of self-reported exercise and the relationship with weight loss in overweight women. *Med Sci Sports Exerc.* 1998; 30: 634–8.

Kierman M, King AC, Stefanick ML, Killen JD. Men gain additional psychological benefits by adding exercise to a weight-loss program. *Obes Res.* 2001; 9: 770–7.

Klem ML, Wing RR, McGuire MT, Seagle HM, Hill J. A descriptive study of individuals successful at long-term weight maintenance of substantial weight loss. *Am J Clin Nutr.* 1997; 66: 239–46.

Lichtman SW, Pisarska K, Berman ER, Pestone M, Dowling H, Offenbacher E, Weisel H, Heshka S, Matthews DE, and Heymsfield SB. Discrepancy between self-reported and actual calorie intake and exercise in obese subjects. *N Eng J Med.* 1992; 327: 1893–8.

Lissner L. Measuring food intake in studies of obesity. *Public Health Nutr.* 2002; 5: 889–92.

McArdle WD, Katch FI, Katch VL. *Sports and Exercise Nutrition*, 2nd ed. Baltimore: Lippincott Williams &Wilkins, 2005.

Permanente Journal Focus on Obesity Part 2: The National Weight Control Registry. Accessed online, October 3, 2006, at http://xnet.kp.org/permanentejournal/sum03/registry.html

Saris WH. Fit, fat and fat free: the metabolic aspects of weight control. In *J Obes Relat Metab Disord.* 1998; 22: S15–21.

2005 Dietary Guidelines Advisory Committee Report. Accessed online October 3, 2006, at www.healthierus.gov/dietaryguidelines/

U.S. Surgeon General. *Physical Activity and Health: A Report of the Surgeon General Executive Summary.* Accessed online October 3, 2006, at www.cdc.gov/nccdphp/sgr/sgr.htm

Chapter 10. Support: Everybody Needs Some

Heshka S, Anderson JW, Atkinson RL, Greenway FL, Hill JO, Phinney SD, Kolotkin RL, Miller-Kovach K, Pi-Sunyer FX. Weight loss with self-help compared with a structured commercial program: a randomized trial. *JAMA.* 2003; 289: 1792–8.

Institute of Medicine. *Weighing the Options: Criteria for Evaluating Weight-Management Programs.* Washington, DC: National Academies Press, 1995.

Ogden J, Taylor C. Dieting and cognitive style: the role of current and past dieting behaviour and cognitions. *J Health Psych 01.* 2000; 5: 17–24.

Position of the American Dietetic Association: weight management. *J Am Diet Assoc.* 2002; 102: 1145–55.

Rippe JM. *Weight Watchers Weight Loss That Lasts.* Hoboken, NJ: John Wiley & Sons, 2005.

Chapter 11. Couples Win the Weight-Loss Race

Barlow SE, Dietz W Jr. Obesity evaluation and treatment: expert committee recommendations. *Pediatrics.* 1998; 102: e29.

Benton D. Role of parents in the determination of the food preferences of children and the development of obesity. *In J Obes Relat Metab Disord.* 2004; 28: 858–69.

Blissett J, Meyer C, Haycraft E. Maternal and paternal controlling feeding practices with male and female children. *Appetite.* 2006; 47: 212–9.

Block KV, Klein CH, de Souza e Silva NA, Nogueira Ada R, Salis LH. Socio-economic aspects of spousal concordance for hypertension, obesity, and smoking in a community of Rio de Janeiro, Brazil. *Arq Bras Cardiol.* 2003; 80: 179–86.

Burke V, Giangiulio N, Gillam HF, Beilin LJ, Houghton S, Milligan RA. Health promotion in couples adapting to a shared lifestyle. *Health Educ Res.* 1999; 14: 269–88.

Burke V, Mori TA, Giangiulio N, Gillam HF, Beilin LJ, Houghton S, Cutt HE, Mansour J, Wilson A. An innovative program for changing health behaviours. *Asia Pac J Clin Nutr.* 2002; 11: S586–97.

Foreyt JP, Ramirez AG, Cousins JH. Cuidando El Corazon—a weight-reduction intervention for Mexican Americans. *Am J Clin Nutr.* 1991; 53: S1639–41.

Fulkerson JA, Story M, Mellin A, Leffert N, Neumark-Sztainer D, French SA. Family dinner meal frequency and adolescent development: relationships with developmental assets and high-risk behaviors. *J Adolesc Health.* 2006; 39: 337–45.

Jeffery RW, Rick AM. Cross-sectional and longitudinal associations between body mass index and marriage-related factors. *Obes Res.* 2002 Aug; 10: 809–15.

Johannsen DL, Johannsen NM, Specker BL. Influence of parents' eating behaviors and child feeding practices on children's weight status. *Obesity.* 2006; 14: 431–9.

Johnson SL, Birch LL. Parents' and children's adiposity and eating style. *Pediatrics.* 1994; 94: 653–61.

Katzmarzyk PT, Perusse L, Rao DC, Bouchard C. Spousal resemblance and risk of 7-year increases in obesity and central adiposity in the Canadian population. *Obes Res.* 1999; 7: 545–51.

Knuiman MW, Divitini ML, Bartholomew HC, Welborn TA. Spouse correlations in cardiovascular risk factors and the effect of marriage duration. *Am J Epidemiol.* 1996; 143: 48–53.

Kratt P, Reynolds K, Shewchuk R. The role of availability as a moderator of family fruit and vegetable consumption. *Health Educ Behav.* 2000; 27: 471–82.

Macken LC, Yates B, Blancher S. Concordance of risk factors in female spouses of male patients with coronary disease. *J Cardiopulm Rehabil.* 2000; 20: 361–8.

Miller-Kovach K. *Weight Watchers Family Power.* Hoboken, NJ: John Wiley & Sons, 2006.

Ogden CL, Carroll MD, Curtin LR, McDowell MA, Tabak CJ, Flegal KM. Prevalence of overweight and obesity in the United States, 1999–2004. *JAMA.* 2006; 295: 1549–55.

Pyke SD, Wood DA, Kinmonth AL, Thompson SG. Change in coronary risk and coronary risk factor levels in couples following lifestyle intervention. The British Family Heart Study. *Arch Fam Med.* 1997; 6: 354–60.

U.S. Surgeon General. *The Surgeon General's Call to Action to Prevent and Decrease Overweight and Obesity.* Accessed online October 6, 2006, at www .surgeongeneral.gov/topics/obesity/

Wardle J, Guthrie C, Sanderson S, Birch L, Plomin R. Food and activity preferences in children of lean and obese parents. *Int J Obes Relat Metab Disord.* 2001; 25: 971–7.

Chapter 12. Living Healthy: Lifestyle Is Key

Coakley EH, Rimm EB, Colditz G, Kawachi I, Willet W. Predictors of weight change in men: results from the Health Professionals Follow-Up Study. *Int J Obes Relat Metab Disord.* 1998; 22: 89–96.

Heshka S, Anderson JW, Atkinson RL, Greenway FL, Hill JO, Phinney SD, Kolotkin RL, Miller-Kovach K, Pi-Sunyer FX. Weight loss with self-help compared with a structured commercial program: a randomized trial. *JAMA.* 2003; 289: 1792–8.

Klem ML, Wing RR, Lang W, McGuire MT, Hill JO. Does weight loss maintenance become easier over time? *Obes Res.* 2000; 8: 438–44.

Kelm ML, Wing RR, McGuire MT, Seagle HM, Hill JO. A descriptive study of individuals successful at long-term weight maintenance of substantial weight loss. *Am J Clin Nutr.* 1998; 67: 239–46.

Klem ML, Wing RR, McGuire MT, Seagle HM, Hill JO. A descriptive study of individuals successful at long-term maintenance of substantial weight loss. *Am J Clin Nutr.* 1998; 67: 946.

Permanente Journal Focus on Obesity Part 2: The National Weight Control Registry. Accessed online, October 3, 2006, at http://xnet.kp.org/permanentejournal/ sum03/registry.html

Shick SM, Wing RR, Klem ML, McGuire MT, Hill JO, Seagle H. Persons successful at long-term weight-loss and maintenance continue to consume a low-energy, low-fat diet. *J Am Diet Assoc.* 1998; 98: 408–13.

2005 Dietary Guidelines Advisory Committee Report. Accessed online October 3, 2006, at www.healthierus.gov/dietaryguidelines/

Wing RR, Jeffery RW. Benefits of recruiting participants with friends and increasing social support for weight loss and maintenance. *J Consult Clin Psychol.* 1999; 67: 132–8.

Wyatt HR, Grunwald GK, Mosca CL, Klem ML, Wing RR, Hill JO. Long-term weight loss and breakfast in subjects in the National Weight Control Registry. *Obes Res.* 2002; 10: 78–82.

Credits

Charts

Page 13: Data from Colditz GA, Willett WC, Rotnitzky A, Manson JE. Weight gain as a risk factor for clinical diabetes mellitus in women. *Ann Intern Med* 1995; 122:481–6.

Page 14: Data from Calle EE, Thun MJ, Petrelli JM, et al. Body-mass index and mortality in a prospective cohort of US adults. *N Engl J Med* 1999; 341:1097–1105.

Page 83: Data from McArdle WD, Katch FI, Katch VL. *Sports and Exercise Nutrition*, 2nd ed. (Philadelphia: Lippincott Williams & Wilkins, 2005.)

Photos

Page 23: John Dyer/NPN Worldwide

Pages 41, 209: Robb Gregg/NPN Worldwide

Pages 61, 97: Michael Paras/NPN Worldwide

Page 78: Stephen Hill/NPN Worldwide

Page 114: David Tejada/NPN Worldwide

Pages 133, 173: Hasnain Dattu/NPN Worldwide

Page 153: John Jernigan/NPN Worldwide

Page 192: Leon Gehar/NPN Worldwide

Index